NCLEX-RN
· ·
FLASH REVIEW

NCLEX-RN
FLASH REVIEW

DR. ALICIA CULLEITON
DR. YVONNE WEIDEMAN

WITHDRAWN

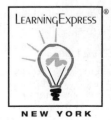

LEARNINGEXPRESS®

NEW YORK

Copyright © 2012 LearningExpress, LLC.
All rights reserved under International and Pan American Copyright Conventions.
Published in the United States by LearningExpress, LLC, New York.

Library of Congress Cataloging-in-Publication Data
NCLEX-RN flash review.—1st ed.
     p. ; cm.
   ISBN 978-1-57685-893-6 (alk. paper)—ISBN 1-57685-893-6 (alk. paper)
   I. LearningExpress (Organization)
   [DNLM: 1. Nursing Care—Examination Questions.   WY 18.2]
   610.73076—dc23

                                                                      2012017106

Printed in the United States of America

9 8 7 6 5 4 3 2 1

First Edition

ISBN 978-1-57685-893-6

For more information or to place an order, contact LearningExpress at:
     2 Rector Street
     26th Floor
     New York, NY 10006

ABOUT THE CONTRIBUTORS

Dr. Yvonne Weideman is an Assistant Professor of Nursing at Duquesne University School of Nursing. Her areas of interest are the preparation of students for the NCLEX exam and the use of innovative technology in the classroom to enhance learning. Dr. Weideman has recently developed a model for integrating theory and content through the use of virtual technology entitled the Virtual Pregnancy Model.

Dr. Alicia Culleiton is an Assistant Clinical Professor at Duquesne University School of Nursing. She currently teaches doctoral-level nursing courses as well as undergraduate NCLEX-RN preparation courses. Dr. Culleiton earned her BSN from the Catholic University of America, her MSN in nursing administration and nursing education from Indiana University of Pennsylvania, and her PhD from Chatham University. She is published in nursing and educational journals. Her clinical expertise is in emergency/trauma and critical care nursing, with research interests in student remediation and NCLEX-RN preparation.

Dr. Karen Paraska Graf, PhD, MSN, CRNP, is assistant professor of nursing at Duquesne University. She has taught a range of graduate nursing courses, including offerings in advanced practice nursing and research methods, as well as undergraduate courses, including NCLEX-RN preparation courses. She is co-author of several referred articles, including "Cognitive impairment associated with adjuvant therapy in breast cancer" for the journal *Psycho-Oncology*.

CONTENTS

About This Book . . . . **xxv**

Part I: General Concepts **1**
Denture Care Procedures 3
Food Sources: Calcium 3
Food Sources: Iron 3
Food Sources: Magnesium 5
Food Sources: Phosphorus 5
Food Sources: Potassium 5
Food Sources: Sodium 7
Laboratory Values, Normal Hematology 7
Laboratory Values, Normal Metabolic 9
Laboratory Values, Normal Renal 9
Mathematical Formulas, Common: Intravenous Therapies 11
Mathematical Formulas, Common: Medication Dosage 11
Medication Administration, Six Rights of 13
Medication Levels, Toxic 13
Medication Suffixes 15
Medications and Antidotes, Common 15
Metric Conversions 17
Metric Abbreviations 17
Nursing Process Steps 17
Vital Signs, Normal 19

Part II: Adult **21**
Section 1: Acid-Base, Fluid, and Electrolyte Imbalances **23**
Acid-Base Imbalances: Signs and Symptoms of 23
Acid-Base Imbalances: Treatment Modalities 23
Arterial Blood Gases (ABG): Terms and Values 25
Arterial Blood Gases (ABG): Fully Compensated ABG Interpretations . . 25
Arterial Blood Gases (ABG): Partially Compensated
  ABG Interpretations 25

Calcium (Ca) Imbalance 27
Hypercalcemia 27
Hyperkalemia. 27
Hypermagnesemia 29
Hypernatremia. 29
Hypocalcemia 29
Hypokalemia 31
Hypomagnesemia 31
Hyponatremia 33
Magnesium (Mg) Imbalance 33
Potassium (K⁺) Imbalance. 33
Sodium (Na) Imbalance 35
Tonicity of IV Fluids. 35

Section 2: Cardiovascular Disorders. 37
Afterload 37
Aneurysm 37
Angina 37
Angina: Types or Patterns of 39
Aortic Insufficiency. 39
Aortic Stenosis 39
Atrial Fibrillation 41
Buerger's Disease (Thromboangiitis Obliterans). 41
Cardiac Output (CO) 41
Catheterization, Cardiac 43
Coronary Angioplasty, Percutaneous Transluminal (PTCA) 43
Coronary Artery Bypass Graft (CABG) 43
Coronary Artery Disease (CAD) 45
Electrocardiogram (ECG): Steps for Interpreting 45
Endocarditis (Bacterial, Infective) 47
Heart Failure 47
Heart Sounds. 49
Hypertension: Classification of. 49
Hypertension Management 51
Insufficiency 51
Intermittent Claudication 51
Medications: Antianginal. 53
Medications: Antihypertensive, I 53
Medications: Antihypertensive, II. 55
Medications: Diuretic. 55
Medications: Nitroglycerin Administration, Client Education for 57
Mitral Insufficiency 57
Mitral Stenosis 57

Myocardial Infarction (MI)....................................... 59
Myocardial Infarction: Cardiac Enzyme Elevation, Post-MI........... 59
Myocardial Infarction: MONA for................................. 61
Pacemaker, Permanent 61
Pacemaker, Permanent: Client Education 63
Pacemaker, Temporary: Invasive Epicardial Pacing 63
Pacemaker, Temporary: Invasive Transvenous Pacing............... 65
Pacemaker, Temporary: Noninvasive Transvenous Pacing............ 65
Pain Assessment: PQRST Method................................. 67
Pericarditis 69
Peripheral Arterial Disease (PAD) 69
Peripheral Arterial Disease: Client Education for................... 71
Phlebitis.. 71
Preload... 71
Pulmonary Edema.. 73
Raynaud's Phenomenon... 73
Shock States 75
Sinus Bradycardia... 77
Sinus Rhythm, Normal 77
Sinus Tachycardia... 79
Stenosis 79
Stroke Volume (SV) 79
Valvular Defects: Comparison of Symptomatology of, I.............. 81
Valvular Defects: Comparison of Symptomatology of, II............. 81
Venous Thrombosis (Thrombophlebitis)........................... 83
Ventricular Contractions/Complexes, Premature (PVCs)............. 83
Ventricular Fibrillation (VF) 85
Ventricular Tachycardia (VT).................................... 85

Section 3: Endocrine Disorders 87
Addison's Crisis... 87
Addison's Disease.. 87
Chvostek's Sign... 87
Cushing's Disease.. 89
Diabetes Insipidus 89
Diabetes Mellitus 89
Diabetes, Type I... 91
Diabetes, Type 2 91
Diabetic Ketoacidosis (DKA).................................... 93
DKA and HHNS, Differences Between 93
Hyperglycemia.. 93
Hyperglycemic Hyperosmolar Nonketotic Syndrome (HHNS).......... 95
Hyperpituitarism.. 95

Hyperthyroidism/Graves' Disease 95
Hypoglycemia 97
Hypopituitarism 97
Hypothyroidism. 97
Insulin, Types of: Intermediate-Acting and Long-Acting 99
Insulin, Types of: Rapid-Acting and Short-Acting 99
Myxedema 101
Somogyi Phenomenon 101
Thyroid Storm 101
Trousseau's Sign 101

Section 4: Eye and Ear Disorders. **103**
Cataracts 103
Ear Drops, Administration of 103
Eyedrops, Administration of 103
Glaucoma 105
Hearing Loss, Types of 105
Hyperopia. 105
Macular Degeneration 107
Mydriasis 107
Myopia 109
Retinal Detachment 109

Section 5: Gastrointestinal Disorders **111**
Ascites 111
Bowel (or Intestinal) Obstruction 111
Cholecystitis 111
Cholelithiasis 113
Cirrhosis 113
Cirrhosis, Types of. 115
Crohn's Disease. 115
Cullen's Sign. 115
Diverticulitis 117
Esophageal Varices. 117
Fector Hepaticus. 117
Gastroesophageal Reflux Disease (GERD) 119
Hepatitis 119
Hepatitis A (HAV) 119
Hepatitis B (HBV) 121
Hepatitis C (HCV) 121
Hiatal Hernia 121
Jaundice. 123
Murphy's Sign 123

Pancreatitis *123*

Peptic Ulcer Disease (PUD) *125*

Peristalsis *125*

Portal Hypertension *125*

Turner's Sign *127*

Ulcerative Colitis *127*

Section 6: Hematological Disorders **129**

Acute Transfusion Reactions *129*

Anemia *129*

Anemia, Aplastic *131*

Anemia, Iron-Deficiency *131*

Anemia, Megaloblastic *133*

Blood Products I *133*

Blood Products II *135*

Intramuscular Medication Administration: Z-Track Method *135*

Leukemia *137*

Polycythemia *137*

Thrombocytopenia *139*

Section 7: Integumentary Disorders **141**

Burns, Causes of *141*

Burns, Chemical: Emergency Management *141*

Burns, Electrical: Emergency Management *141*

Burns, Thermal: Emergency Management *143*

Burn Depth I *143*

Burn Depth II *145*

Fluid Resuscitation Formulas: First 24 Hours Following a Burn Injury. *145*

Herpes Zoster (Shingles) *147*

Inhalation Injury: Emergency Management *147*

Pressure Ulcers, Stages of *149*

Rule of Nines *149*

Section 8: Musculoskeletal Disorders **151**

Amputation *151*

Crutch Walking *151*

Crutch Walking: Going Up Stairs *151*

Fracture *153*

Fractures, Complications of, I *153*

Fractures, Complications of, II *153*

Fractures, Hip, Femoral Neck *155*

Fractures, Hip, Intertrochanteric *155*

Fractures, Types of *157*

Gout *157*

Osteomyelitis 159
Osteoporosis 159
Reduction, Types of. 161
Rheumatoid Arthritis 161
Traction: General Nursing Care 163
Traction, Skeletal 163
Traction, Skin. 163
Traction, Types of 165

Section 9: Neurological Disorders. 167
Agnosia. 167
Alexia 167
Apraxia 167
Autonomic Dysreflexia 169
Babinski Reflex 169
Bell's Palsy 169
Brudinski Reflex 171
Caloric Testing. 171
Cerebral Perfusion Pressure (CPP), Calculation of. 171
Cerebral Spinal Fluid, Recognition/Testing for 173
Cranial Nerves 173
Craniotomy. 173
Craniotomy, Postoperative Care 175
Decorticate and Decerebrate Posturing 175
Dysarthria 175
Dysphagia 177
Dysphasia. 177
Flaccid Posturing 177
Glasgow Coma Scale. 179
Guillain-Barré Syndrome 179
Head Injury 181
Head Injury, Client Education Discharge Instructions 181
Head Injury, Types of, I. 183
Head Injury, Types of, II 183
Hemianopsia 185
Homonymous Hemianopsia 185
Increased Intracranial Pressure (ICP) 185
Kernig's Sign 187
Mean Arterial Pressure (MAP), Calculation for 187
Meningeal Irritation, Signs and Symptoms of 187
Meningitis 189
Multiple Sclerosis (MS) 189

Myasthenia Gravis 191
Nuchal Rigidity 191
Oculocephalic Reflex (Doll's Eye Reflex) 191
Parkinson's Disease 193
Respiratory Patterns, Abnormal 193
Seizure 195
Seizure, Types of: Generalized Seizures, I 195
Seizure, Types of: Generalized Seizures, II 197
Spinal Cord Injury (SCI) 197
Spinal Cord Injury, Specific Assessment Findings 199
Spinal Shock 199
Spinal Shock and Autonomic Dysreflexia, Differences Between 199
Stroke, Manifestations of 201
Stroke or Cerebral Vascular Accident (CVA) 201
Tetraplegia and Paraplegia 201

Section 10: Oncology Disorders 203
Breast Cancer 203
Breast Self-Examination (BSE), Instructions for 203
Lung Cancer 205
Metastasis: Common Sites 205
Testicular Cancer 207
Testicular Self-Examination, Instructions for 207

Section 11: Renal Disorders 209
Arterial Steal Syndrome 209
Azotemia 209
Continuous Renal Replacement Therapy (CRRT) 209
Creatinine Clearance Test 211
Cystitis 211
Dialysis, Vascular Access for 211
Diet, Acid-Ash 213
Diet, Alkaline-Ash 213
Diet, Food Sources High in Purine, Calcium, and Oxalate 213
Glomerular Filtration Rate (GFR) 215
Glomerulonephritis 215
Hemodialysis 215
Hemodialysis, Complications of 217
Peritoneal Dialysis 217
Peritoneal Dialysis, Complications of 217
Peritoneal Dialysis, Continuous Ambulatory 219
Pyelonephritis 219

Renal Failure, Acute (ARF)....................................... 219
Renal Failure, Acute, Causes of 221
Renal Failure, Acute, Clinical Manifestations of 221
Renal Failure, Acute, Management of 223
Renal Failure, Acute, Phases of 225
Renal Failure, Chronic (CRF) 227
Renal Failure, Chronic, Management of 227
Renal Failure, Chronic: Stage 1, Diminished Renal Reserve.......... 227
Renal Failure, Chronic: Stage 2, Renal Insufficiency 229
Renal Failure, Chronic: Stage 3, End-Stage Renal Failure 229
Risk Factors: Intrarenal Failure (Kidney Tissue Disease) 231
Risk Factors: Postrenal Failure (Obstructive Problems)............. 231
Risk Factors: Prerenal Failure (Renal Ischemia)................... 231
Specific Gravity 233
Urinary/Renal Calculi 233
Urinary/Renal Calculi, Dietary and Medical Management of 235
Urinary/Renal Calculi, Major Categories of 235
Urinary System: Common Abnormalities Assessment I 237
Urinary System: Common Abnormalities Assessment II............ 237
Urinary Tract Infection (UTI) 239

Section 12: Respiratory Disorders............................. 241
Acute Respiratory Distress Syndrome (ARDS)..................... 241
Asthma.. 241
Breath Sounds... 243
Bronchitis, Chronic... 245
Chest Physiotherapy (CPT) Procedure........................... 245
Congestive Obstructive Pulmonary Disease (COPD) 247
Emphysema 247
Hemothorax... 249
Incentive Spirometry, Client Instructions for 249
Legionnaires' Disease 249
Lung Cancer 251
Mechanical Ventilation, Controls and Settings, I.................. 251
Mechanical Ventilation, Controls and Settings, II 253
Mechanical Ventilation, Modes of 255
Pneumonia... 255
Pneumothorax 257
Pulmonary Embolism (PE)...................................... 257
Tuberculosis (TB) 259
Tuberculosis, Client Education for 259
Tuberculosis, Risk Factors/Causes of........................... 261

Part III: Obstetrics **263**

Section 1: Antepartum **265**

Ballottement 265

Bishop Score 265

Braxton Hicks Contractions 265

Chadwick's Sign 267

Goodell's Sign 267

GTPAL 267

Hegar's Sign 269

Morning Sickness/Hyperemesis Gravidarum 269

Naegele's Rule 269

Nutrition 271

Prenatal Visits 271

Psychosocial Tasks 271

Quickening 273

Rh Incompatibility 273

Signs of Pregnancy 273

System, Cardiovascular 275

System, Gastrointestinal 275

System, Genitourinary 275

System, Integumentary 277

System, Musculoskeletal 277

System, Respiratory 277

Weight Gain 279

Weight Gain Distribution 279

Section 2: Intrapartum **281**

Amniotic Fluid Characteristics 281

Cardinal Movements of Labor 281

Cervical Dilation 281

Cervical Effacement 283

Cesarean Delivery 283

Pain Relief: Nonpharmacological 283

Pain Relief: Pharmacological 285

Passageway 285

Passenger 285

Powers of Labor 287

Psyche 287

Signs of Impending Labor 287

Stage of Labor, First 289

Stage of Labor, Second 289

Stage of Labor, Third 289

Stage of Labor, Fourth 291
Station 291
Timing Contractions 291
True versus False Labor 293

Section 3: Postpartum..................................... **295**
Assessment/Nursing Interventions in Postpartum Period.......... 295
Bonding Phases (Rubin's) 295
Fundal Assessment... 295
Lochia 297

Section 4: Maternal Complications, Antepartum **299**
Abruptio Placenta... 299
Anemia 299
Disseminated Intravascular Coagulation (DIC)................... 299
Eclampsia... 301
Ectopic Pregnancy 301
Gestational Diabetes 301
Gestational Hypertension 303
HELLP Syndrome 303
Hydatidiform Mole 303
Hyperemesis Gravidarum...................................... 305
Incompetent Cervix.. 305
Placenta Previa 305
Preeclampsia.. 307
Preterm Labor 307

Section 5: Maternal Complications, Intrapartum **309**
Amniotic Fluid Embolism 309
Dystocia 309
Fetal Distress 309
Fetal Demise 311
Inverted Uterus 311
Precipitate Labor.. 311
Premature Rupture of Membranes (PROM) 313
Uterine Rupture... 313

Section 6: Maternal Complications, Postpartum **315**
Mastitis 315
Postpartum Depression....................................... 315
Postpartum Hemorrhage....................................... 315
Puerperal Infection.. 317
Uterine Atony... 317

Section 7: Maternal Medication *319*
Antenatal Corticosteroids *319*
Ergot Alkaloids *319*
Magnesium Sulfate... *319*
Opioids *321*
Prostaglandins *321*
RhoGAM *321*
Tocolytics *323*
Uterine Stimulants *323*

Section 8: Fetal Development............................... *325*
Month 1.. *325*
Month 2 .... *325*
Month 3 .... *325*
Month 4 .... *327*
Month 5 .... *327*
Month 6 .... *327*
Month 7 .... *329*
Month 8 .... *329*
Month 9 .... *329*
Fetal Circulation *331*

Section 9: Fetal Assessment................................ *333*
Fetal Heart Rate Acceleration *333*
Fetal Heart Rate: Early Deceleration *333*
Fetal Heart Rate: Late Deceleration *333*
Fetal Heart Rate Variability................................... *335*
Fetal Heart Tones *335*
Fundal Height *335*
Leopold Maneuvers... *337*

Section 10: Neonate Assessment............................ *339*
Acrocyanosis *339*
Apgar Score *339*
Caput Succedaneum *339*
Cephalhematoma *341*
Epstein Pearls *341*
Fontanels.. *341*
Harlequin Color Changes *343*
Head Lag... *343*
Head to Toe: HEENT/Neurological............................. *343*
Head to Toe: Head-to-Chest Ratio *345*
Head to Toe: Heart and Lungs................................. *345*

Head to Toe: Abdomen/Genitalia/Spine/Extremities 345
Lanugo 347
Meconium.. 347
Milia 347
Molding 349
Mongolian Spots... 349
Reflexes 349
Vernix Caseosa 351

Section 11: Neonate Care 353
Breast-Feeding Tips 353
Circumcision Care 353
Umbilical Cord 353

Section 12: Neonate Complications............................ 355
Drug-Dependent Neonate 355
Fetal Alcohol Syndrome 355
Hyperbilirubinemia 355
Hypoglycemia 357
Meconium Aspiration 357
Preterm Neonate... 357
Respiratory Distress Syndrome 359

Section 13: Neonate Medications 361
Eye Prophylaxis... 361
Lung Surfactants.. 361

Part IV: Pediatrics, General 363
Section 1: Growth and Development........................... 365
Developmental Periods 365
Direction of Growth 365
Theorists: Erik Erikson................................... 365
Theorists: Sigmund Freud 367
Theorists: Lawrence Kohlberg.............................. 367
Theorists: Jean Piaget 367

Section 2: Developmental Milestones 369
Infant: Fine/Gross Motor.................................. 369
Infant: Language/Cognitive/Social......................... 369
Toddler: Fine/Gross Motor................................. 369
Toddler: Language/Cognitive/Social........................ 371
Preschoolers 371
Play.. 371

Section 3: Assessment **373**
Abdomen/Genitalia 373
Head/Eyes/Ears/Nose/Mouth 373
Musculature 373
Neurological: Reflexes 375
Skin 375
Teeth/ Chest/Heart/ Lungs 375
Vaccination Schedule, Ages 0 to 6, for All 377
Vaccination Schedule, Ages 7 to 18, for All 377

Part V: Pediatrics, Disorders **379**
Section 1: Abuse **381**
Child Abuse: General 381
Child Abuse: Types 381

Section 2: Cardiovascular Disorders **383**
Aortic Stenosis 383
Atrial Septal Defect 383
Coarctation of Aorta 383
Congestive Heart Failure 385
Hypoplastic Left-Heart Syndrome . . . . : 385
Jones Criteria 385
Patent Ductus Arteriosus 387
Pulmonary Artery Stenosis 387
Rheumatic Heart Disease (RHD)/Rheumatic Fever (RF) 387
Tetralogy of Fallot 389
Transposition of Great Vessels 389
Truncus Arteriosis 389
Ventral Septal Defect (VSD) 391

Section 3: Endocrine Disorders **393**
Dehydration 393
Diabetes Mellitus 393
Fever 393
Phenylketonuria 395

Section 4: Gastrointestinal Disorders **397**
Appendicitis 397
Celiac Disease 397
Cleft Lip/Palate 397
Esophageal Atresia/Tracheoesophageal Fistula 399
Hirschsprung's Disease 399
Intestinal Parasites: Giardiasis 399

Intestinal Parasites: Pinworms.................................. 401
Intussusceptions 401
Omphalocele 401
Poisoning... 403
Poisoning: Aspirin/Acetaminophen/Corrosives 403
Poisoning: Lead... 405
Pyloric Stenosis.. 405
Vomiting/Diarrhea 407

Section 5: Genitourinary Disorders 409
Cryptorchidism 409
Enuresis 409
Epispadias/Hypospadias 409
Glomerulonephritis 411
Urinary Tract Infection....................................... 411

Section 6: Head, Eye, Ear Disorders 413
Conjunctivitis (Pink Eye) 413
Otitis Media.. 413
Pediculosis (Lice) 413

Section 7: Hematological/Immune System Disorders 415
Allergies... 415
Hemophilia.. 415
Leukemia 417
Sickle-Cell Anemia.. 417

Section 8: Integumentary Disorders 419
Acne Vulgaris (Acne) 419
Dermatitis/Diaper Rash.. 419
Eczema 419
Impetigo.. 421

Section 9: Musculoskeletal Disorders 423
Barlow Maneuver 423
Hip Dysplasia... 423
Juvenile Rheumatoid Arthritis 423
Muscular Dystrophy (Duchenne's)............................... 425
Ortolanti's Maneuver 425
Scoliosis... 425

Section 10: Neurological/Cognitive Disorders 427
Attention-Deficit/Hyperactivity Disorder (ADHD) 427
Autism 427
Cerebral Palsy 429

Cerebral Palsy: Types 429

Hydrocephalus.. 431

Neural Tube Defects 431

Reye's Syndrome 433

Spina Bifida 433

Spina Bifida: Types/Symptoms 433

Trisomy 21 (Down Syndrome) 435

Section 11: Respiratory Disorders **437**

Asthma... 437

Bronchopulmonary Dysplasia.................................... 437

Croup (Laryngotracheobronchitis)............................... 437

Cystic Fibrosis... 439

Epiglottitis.. 439

Respiratory Syncytial Virus (RSV)/Bronchiolitis 439

Sudden Infant Death Syndrome (SIDS) 441

Sudden Infant Death Syndrome (SIDS) Risk Reduction............ 441

Part VI: Pediatrics, Medication.............................. **443**

Calculations.. 445

Intramuscular Injections 445

Intravenous Burette Sets....................................... 445

Metered Dose Inhalers, Administration of 447

Nasal Drops/Otic Drops, Administration of....................... 447

Oral Medications, Administration of 447

Subcutaneous Injections....................................... 449

Part VII: Mental Health..................................... **451**

Section 1: Anxiety Disorders................................. **453**

Anxiety... 453

Anxiety: Generalized... 453

Obsessive-Compulsive Disorder 455

Panic Disorder.. 455

Phobia.. 457

Post-Traumatic Stress Disorder 457

Section 2: Cognitive Disorders............................... **459**

Alzheimer's Disease 459

Amnestic Disorders 459

Delirium 459

Vascular Dementia 461

Section 3: Delusional Disorders.............................. **463**

Delusional Disorders, General.................................. 463

Delusional Disorders, Types of 463

Section 4: Dissociative Disorders 465
Depersonalization Disorder. 465
Dissociative Amnesia 465
Dissociative Identity Disorder. 465

Section 5: Eating Disorders 467
Anorexia Nervosa 467
Bulimia Nervosa 467

Section 6: Mood Disorders 469
Bipolar Disorder 469
Depression. 469
Suicide 471

Section 7: Personality Disorders. 473
Antisocial Personality Disorder 473
Borderline Personality Disorder. 473
Dependent Personality Disorder. 473
Paranoid Personality Disorder 475

Section 8: Schizophrenia Disorders 477
Schizophrenia Disorders, Overview/General Principles 477
Catatonic Schizophrenia 477
Disorganized Schizophrenia 477
Paranoid Schizophrenia 479

Section 9: Sexual Disorders 481
Gender Dysphoria 481
Paraphilias 481
Sexual Dysfunction 481
Sexual Dysfunction, Types of 483

Section 10: Somatoform Disorders 485
Somatoform Disorders, Overview/General Principles 485
Body Dysmorphic Disorder 485
Conversion Disorder 485
Hypochondria 487
Pain Disorder. 487
Somatization Disorder 487

Section 11: Substance Abuse 489
Alcohol Dependency/Abuse. 489
Alcohol: Korsakoff's Psychosis 489
Alcohol: Wernicke's Encephalopathy 489
Alcohol: Withdrawal 491

CAGE Questionnaire *491*

Non-Alcohol Substance Abuse *491*

Substance: Cocaine. *493*

Substance: Hallucinogenic. *493*

Substance: Narcotics/Opioids *493*

Substance: Sedatives *495*

Substance: Stimulants *495*

Substance Abuse, Important Terminology *495*

Section 12: Therapeutic Communication **497**

Therapeutic Communication, Phases of *497*

Therapeutic Communication Techniques, I *497*

Therapeutic Communication Techniques, II. *499*

Section 13: Therapies **501**

Behavioral Therapy. *501*

Cognitive Therapy. *501*

Crisis Intervention *501*

Family Therapy. *503*

Group Therapy. *503*

Milieu Therapy. *503*

Section 14: Medications. **505**

Acetylcholinesterone Inhibitors *505*

Antiparkinson *505*

Antipsychotic. *505*

Anti-Substance Abuse *507*

Atypical Antidepressants. *507*

Barbiturates/Sedatives *507*

Benzodiazepines. *509*

Monoamine Oxidase Inhibitors (MAOIs) *509*

Mood Stabilizers/Antimanic *511*

Selective Serotonin Reuptake Inhibitors (SSRIs) *511*

Tricyclic Antidepressants. *513*

Additional Online Practice **515**

ABOUT THIS BOOK

This book contains more than 600 terms and concepts that most commonly show up on the National Council Licensure Examination for Registered Nurses (NCLEX-RN). The terms are divided into seven major parts: General Concepts, Adult, Obstetrics, Pediatrics (General), Pediatric Disorders, Pediatric Medication, and Mental Health.

This on-the-go, quick review study tool for the NCLEX-RN tests you in the same way that the actual exam does—it goes beyond rote facts and definitions to delve into actual nursing processes. For example, a disease is listed on one side, and then along with the definition of the disease (which you can also find in your course books), the back features causes, symptoms, diagnostics, treatment modalities, and pharmacology.

Each page of this book features two or three terms on the front, with the explanation and application for each on the back. This is a *lot* of information—do not try to learn all 600+ concepts in this book at once! The best approach is to study the words in sets of about 12 to 15 words (four or five pages) each day. Following is a suggested program of study:

- Review a set of terms in the morning. Say each term aloud. Read the explanations aloud, as well. Try to say each explanation in your own words after reading it several times.
- Write the terms down on a sheet of paper, and keep the sheet with you, checking it throughout the day to familiarize yourself with the list.
- In the evening, quiz yourself on the terms. Make a check mark next to the terms and processes you define correctly. The next day, review the terms you were unable to define, and study 12 to 15 new words.
- Periodically quiz yourself on the terms you have already studied to check that you have learned them thoroughly.

Best of luck on your NCLEX-RN study plan and exam!

GENERAL CONCEPTS

DENTURE CARE PROCEDURES

· ·

FOOD SOURCES: CALCIUM

· ·

FOOD SOURCES: IRON

1. Apply gloves.
2. Dentures are fragile; be sure to set a towel (or something soft) over the work area.
3. If the client is able, let him or her remove his or her own dentures.
4. If assistance from the nurse is required, grasp the upper plate at the front teeth and move the dentures up and down to release the suction.
5. Lift the lower plate up on one side at a time.
6. Use warm water to clean dentures.
7. Do not soak dentures for an extended time period.
8. The dentures may have sharp edges; handle carefully.
9. Check the oral cavity (report any abnormalities).
10. Replace the dentures in the client's mouth.
11. If the dentures are to be stored, assure that they are properly labeled with the client's name.

. . . .

Broccoli
Carrots
Cheese
Collard greens
Green beans
Milk
Rhubarb
Spinach
Tofu
Yogurt

. . . .

Dark-green leafy vegetables
Egg yolk
Fortified breads and cereals
Liver
Meats

FOOD SOURCES: MAGNESIUM

. . . .

FOOD SOURCES: PHOSPHORUS

. . . .

FOOD SOURCES: POTASSIUM

Avocado
Cauliflower
Green leafy vegetables
Legumes (beans and peas)
Milk
Peanut butter
Pork, beef, chicken
Potatoes
Raisins
Rolled cooked oats
White tuna (canned)
Yogurt

· ·

Fish
Nuts
Organ meats
Pork, beef, chicken
Whole grain breads and cereals

· ·

Avocado
Bananas
Cantaloupe
Carrots
Fish
Mushrooms
Pork, beef, chicken
Potatoes
Raisins
Spinach
Strawberries
Tomatoes

FOOD SOURCES: SODIUM

. . . .

LABORATORY VALUES, NORMAL HEMATOLOGY

. . . .

American cheese
Bacon
Butter
Canned food
Cottage cheese
Cured pork
Hot dogs
Ketchup
Lunch meat
Milk
Mustard
Processed food
Snack food
Soy sauce
Table salt
White and whole wheat bread

Red Blood Cell (RBC) Count	♂ 4.7–6.1 millions/μL
	♀ 4.2–5.4 millions/mm^3
Hemoglobin (Hgb)	♂ 14–18 g/dL
	♀ 12–16 g/dL
Hematocrit (Hct)	♂ 42%–52%
	♀ 37%–47%
Mean Corpuscular Hemoglobin (MCH)	27–31 pg/cell
Mean Corpuscular Hemoglobin Concentration (MCHC)	32–36 g/dL of cells
Mean Corpuscular Volume (MCV)	80–90 fL
White Blood Cell (WBC) Count	5,000–10,000 mm^3
Neutrophils	54%–75%
Monocytes	2%–8%
Lymphocytes	25%–40%
Eosinophils	1%–5%
Basophils	0%–1%
Bands	0%–5%
Platelets	150,000–400,000 mm^3

LABORATORY VALUES, NORMAL METABOLIC

· ·

LABORATORY VALUES, NORMAL RENAL

· ·

Albumin	3.5–5.0 g/dL
Alkaline Phosphate	30–120 IU/L
Aspartate Aminotransferase (AST/SGOT)	0–35 IU/L
Alanine Aminotransferase (ALT/SGPT)	4–36 IU/L
Bilirubin (total)	0.3–1 mg/dL
Calcium	9–10 mg/dL
Carbon Dioxide	22–31 mmol/L
Chloride	98–106 mEq/L
Glucose	70–100 mg/dL
Potassium	3.5–5 mEq/L
Protein (total)	6.4–8.3 g/dL
Sodium	136–145 mEq/L

Serum Blood Test	Normal Value
Blood Urea Nitrogen (BUN) Level	8–25 mg/dL
Serum Creatinine Level	0.6–1.3 mg/dL
Serum Uric Acid Level	2.5–8.0 mg/dL
Creatinine Clearance	Male: 97 to 137 ml/min. Female: 88 to 128 ml/min.

MATHEMATICAL FORMULAS, COMMON: INTRAVENOUS THERAPIES

• •

MATHEMATICAL FORMULAS, COMMON: MEDICATION DOSAGE

• •

Intravenous Therapies: Calculating Milliliters per Hour

$$\frac{\text{Total volume to infuse (mL)}}{\text{Total time (hours)}} = \text{mL/hr.}$$

Intravenous Therapies: Calculating Milliliters per Hour When Time Is Less Than One Hour

$$\frac{\text{Total volume}}{\text{Total time (min.)}} = x(\text{ml/min.}) \times 60 \text{ min./hr.} = x(\text{mL/hr.})$$

Intravenous Therapies: Calculating Drops Per Minute

$$\frac{\text{Total volume} \times \text{Drop factor*}}{\text{Total time (min.)}} = \text{Drops per minute (gtt/min.)}$$

*Check tubing package; drop factor may be 10, 15, 20 (macrodrip), or 60 (microdrip) gtt/mL.

· ·

Formula for Calculating a Medication Dosage

$$\frac{\text{D (desired amount)}}{\text{H (have available)}} \times Q \text{ (quantity)} = x \text{ (amount to give)}$$

D (desired amount) is the dosage that the physician has ordered.
H (have available) is the dosage strength as stated on the label of medication.
Q (quantity) is the volume or form in which the dosage strength is available (tablets, capsules, or milliliters).

· ·

PART I

MEDICATION ADMINISTRATION, SIX RIGHTS OF

· ·

MEDICATION LEVELS, TOXIC

· ·

1. Right medication
2. Right route
3. Right time
4. Right client
5. Right dosage
6. Right documentation

· ·

Medication	Normal Value*	Toxic Level*	Signs and Symptoms of Toxicity
Digoxin (Lanoxin)	0.8–2.0 ng/mL	≥ 2.4 ng/mL	Slow or irregular pulse; rapid weight gain; loss of appetite; nausea; vomiting; blurred or yellow vision; unusual tiredness and weakness; swelling of the ankles, legs, or fingers; difficulty breathing
Lidocaine	1.0–5.0 mcg/mL (antiarrhythmic use)	≥ 5.0 mcg/mL	Drowsiness, dizziness, numbness, double vision, nausea, vomiting
Lithium	0.8–1.5 mEq/L	≥ 1.2 mEq/L	*Mild:* Fine hand tremors, polyuria, thirst, nausea *Moderate:* Headache, confusion, weakness, fatigue *Severe:* Dysrhythmias, bradycardia, irregular pulse
Phenytoin (Dilantin)	10–20 mcg/mL	≥ 30 mcg/mL	Rash, severe nausea or vomiting, drowsiness, slurred speech, impaired coordination (ataxia), swollen glands, yellowish discoloration of skin or eyes, joint pain, fever, unusual bleeding, persistent headache
Theophylline	10–20 mcg/mL	≥ 20 mcg/ml	*Mild/moderate, due to rapid infusion:* Hypotension, hyperventilation, tachycardia *Severe:* Seizures, severe dysrhythmias, cardiovascular collapse

*ng = nanograms

· ·

MEDICATION SUFFIXES

. . . .

MEDICATIONS AND ANTIDOTES, COMMON

. . . .

Suffix	Medication Class
-caine	Local anesthetics
-cillin	Penicillins
-dine	H_2 blockers (anti-ulcer)
-done	Opiod analgesics
-ide	Oral hypoglycemics
-lam	Anti-anxiety agents
-micin, -mycin	Antibiotics
-mide	Diuretics
-nium	Neuromuscular agents
-olol	Beta-blockers
-oxacin	Antibiotics
-pam	Anti-anxiety agents
-pril	Ace inhibitors
-sone	Steroids
-statin	Antihyperlipidemics
-vir	Antivirals
-zide	Diuretics

· ·

Medication	Antidote
Acetaminophen	Mucomyst (N-acetylcysteine)
Anticholinergics	Physostigmine (Antilirium)
Anticoagulants	Protamine/Vitamin K
Benzodiazepines	Flumazenial (Romazicon)
Calcium channel blockers	Calcium chloride
Digoxin	Digoxin immune Fab (Digibind)
Heparin	Protamine sulfate
Insulin-induced hypoglycemia	Glucagon
Iron	Deferoxamine (Desferal)
Lead	Edetate calcium disodium (calcium disodium EDTA)
Opiates	Naloxone (Narcan)

· ·

METRIC CONVERSIONS

. . . .

METRIC ABBREVIATIONS

. . . .

NURSING PROCESS STEPS

GENERAL CONCEPTS

Volume	Weight
1 tsp = 5 mL	1 mg = 1,000 µg or 0.001 g
1 tbsp = 15 mL	1 g = 1,000 mg
1 oz = 30 mL	1 gr = 60 mg
1 cup (8 oz.) = 240 mL	1 kg = 2.2 lb or 1 kg = 1,000 g
1 soda can (12 oz.) = 360 mL	1 L of water = 1 kg
1 pint = 480 mL	1 mcg = 0.000001 g
1 quart = 960 mL	1 mL = 0.001 L

Abbreviations
Meter = m
Liter = L
Milliliter = mL
Kilogram = kg
Gram = g
Milligram = mg
Microgram = mcg or µg

Assessment	Analysis	Planning	Implementation	Evaluation
• Assess for symptoms of the disease (subjective data) and signs of the disease (objective data).	• Interpret signs and symptoms. • Identify the client's needs and formulate an appropriate nursing diagnosis.	• Prioritize the nursing diagnosis. • Develop a nursing plan of care with clear goals.	• Provide appropriate nursing care and implement nursing procedures as directed. • Educate the client in relation to his or her specific healthcare needs.	• Evaluate client outcomes compared with those expected. • Modify plan of care if necessary. • Evaluate client's understanding and ability to complete self-care.

VITAL SIGNS, NORMAL

Age	Temperature (°F)	Pulse Rate (beats/minute)	Respiratory Rate (beats/minute)	Blood Pressure (mm Hg)
Neonate	98.6°–99.8°	110–160	30–50	70–72/45–48
1 month– 3 years	98.5°–99.5°	80–130	20–30	90–100/55–63
6–10 years	97.5°–98.6°	75–115	17–25	96–110/57–72
16 years	97.6°–98.6°	55–100	15–20	120–123/76–80
Adult	96.8°–98.6°	50–95	15–20	120/80
Elderly (70+ years)	96.5°–97.5°	55–95	15–20	120/80

Part II

ADULT

PART II

ACID-BASE IMBALANCES: SIGNS AND SYMPTOMS OF

. . . .

ACID-BASE IMBALANCES: TREATMENT MODALITIES

. . . .

Acid-Base Imbalance	Signs and Symptoms
Respiratory Acidosis	Dyspnea, rapid and shallow breathing pattern, respiratory distress, headache, restlessness, altered mental state, seizures, drowsiness, lethargy, coma, papilledema, hypotension, tachycardia, dysrhythmia, warm and flushed skin, diaphoretic
Metabolic Acidosis	Restlessness, drowsiness, headache, confusion, stupor, coma, hypotension, dysrhythmia, cold and clammy skin, shock, nausea, vomiting, Kussmaul respirations
Respiratory Alkalosis	Lightheadedness, inability to concentrate, loss of consciousness, parasthesia, tinnitus, palpitations, tachycardia, dysrhythmia, syncope
Metabolic Alkalosis	Dizziness, weakness, lethargy, coma, seizures, muscle twitching, muscle cramps, parasthesia, dysrhythmia, decreased gastric motility, paralytic ileus

Acid-Base Imbalance	Treatment
Respiratory Acidosis	• Administer bronchodilators, detergents, antibiotics, sodium bicarbonate, sodium lactate intravenously (IV), Ringer's lactate IV, and potassium as ordered. • Suction as indicated, turn and reposition every two hours, implement pulmonary toileting measures, hydrate client, monitor vital signs, and assess arterial blood gases.
Metabolic Acidosis	• Administer sodium bicarbonate, sodium lactate, and lactated Ringer's IV. • If ketoacidosis is present, administer insulin, monitor laboratory values, observe for signs of hyperkalemia, and record intake and output.
Respiratory Alkalosis	• Eliminate causes of hyperventilation, use rebreathing bag, and provide sedation as ordered. Monitor lab values (especially potassium and HCO_3^-).
Metabolic Alkalosis	• Administer acetazolamide (Diamox), IV solution of added electrolytes, and potassium chloride (to clients on long-term diuretic therapy). • Maintain a diet high in potassium, observe for signs of hypokalemia, and record intake and output.

ARTERIAL BLOOD GASES (ABG): TERMS AND VALUES

· ·

ARTERIAL BLOOD GASES (ABG): FULLY COMPENSATED ABG INTERPRETATIONS

· ·

ARTERIAL BLOOD GASES (ABG): PARTIALLY COMPENSATED ABG INTERPRETATIONS

CO_2	Carbon dioxide
H^+	Hydrogen ion
HCO_3^-	Bicarbonate
H_2CO_3	Carbonic acid
O_2	Oxygen
P_{CO_2}	Partial pressure of carbon dioxide
P_{O_2}	Partial pressure of oxygen
S_{O_2}	Arterial oxygen saturation
pH	7.35–7.45
P_{CO_2}	35–45 mmHg
HCO_3^-	22–26 mEq/L
P_{O_2}	80–100 mmHg

. . . .

Imbalance	pH	PaCO$_2$	HCO$_3^-$
Respiratory Acidosis	Normal (↓7.40)	↑	↑
Respiratory Alkalosis	Normal (↑7.40)	↓	↓
Metabolic Acidosis	Normal (↓7.40)	↓	↓
Metabolic Alkalosis	Normal (↑7.40)	↑	↑

. . . .

Imbalance	pH	PaCO$_2$	HCO$_3^-$
Respiratory Acidosis	↓	↑	↑
Respiratory Alkalosis	↑	↓	↓
Metabolic Acidosis	↓	↓	↓
Metabolic Alkalosis	↑	↑	↑

CALCIUM (Ca) IMBALANCE

. . . .

HYPERCALCEMIA

PART II

. . . .

HYPERKALEMIA

Normal Serum Value	General Information
4.3–5.3 mEq/L 9–11 mg/dL	Plays a major role in blood coagulation, cardiac muscle function, and muscle and nerve function.

· ·

Definition: Excessive calcium in the extracellular fluid (serum level greater than 5.3 mEq/L).
Causes: Immobilization, thyrotoxicosis, Paget's disease, excessive intake of vitamin D or calcium supplements, hyperparathyroidism, neoplasm of the thyroid.
Assessment Findings: Nausea, vomiting, anorexia, flank pain, bone pain, decreased muscle tone, pathological fractures, lethargy, weight loss, polydipsia, polyuria, dehydration, stupor, coma. *ECG changes:* shortened QT segments, ventricular dysrhythmias.
Treatment/Nursing Interventions: Treat the underlying cause; immediate reversal can be obtained through the administration of sodium salts IV and diuretics, as prescribed.

· ·

Definition: Excess concentration of potassium ions in extracellular fluid (serum level greater than 5.5 mEq/L).
Causes: Renal disease (inability to excrete potassium), burns, crush injuries, adrenal insufficiency, respiratory or metabolic acidosis, excess potassium administration.
Assessment Findings: Weakness, muscle cramps, flaccid paralysis, irritability, hyperreflexia proceeding to paralysis, bradycardia, dysrhythmia, ventricular fibrillation. *ECG changes:* Elevated or tented T waves, widened QRS complexes, prolonged P-R interval, flattened P waves with depressed S-T segments.
Treatment/Nursing Interventions: Administer diuretics, hypertonic IV glucose with insulin, Kayexalate, IV calcium as prescribed. If acidosis is present, treat with sodium bicarbonate and withhold foods and medications containing potassium.

HYPERMAGNESEMIA

. . . .

HYPERNATREMIA

. . . .

HYPOCALCEMIA

Definition: Excess of magnesium as a result of renal insufficiency or inability to excrete magnesium absorbed from the diet (serum level greater than 2.1 mEq/L).

Causes: Renal insufficiency, overdose of magnesium, severe dehydration, oliguria, excessive usage/overdose of antacids containing magnesium.

Assessment Findings: Hypotension, decreased respirations, sedation, warm sensation in body, bradycardia, cardiac dysrhythmia, hypoactive deep tendon reflexes.

Treatment/Nursing Interventions: Administer calcium gluconate IV slowly via a peripheral vein; monitor vital signs and neurological status.

. . . .

Definition: High concentration of sodium in extracellular fluid (serum level higher than 145 mEq/L).

Causes: Severe diarrhea, decreased water intake, febrile states, ingestion of sodium chloride, excessive loss of water through rapid and deep respiration, renal failure, diabetes insipidus.

Assessment Findings: Weakness, restlessness, delirium, irritability, confusion, hyperpnea, oliguria, increased temperature and pulse, flushed skin, dry mucous membranes, abdominal cramps, convulsions, nausea, anorexia.

Treatment/Nursing Interventions: Record intake and output, restrict sodium in diet, weigh daily, observe vital signs, administer fluids via IV and/or orally, as prescribed.

Special Considerations: If hypernatremia is caused by dehydration, in which fluid is lost and the concentration of ions increases, signs and symptoms will include concentrated urine, oliguria, dry mucous membranes, dry swollen tongue, seizures, coma, flushed skin, increased temperature, tachycardia, and hypertension.

. . . .

Definition: Deficit of calcium in extracellular fluid (serum level lower than 8.5 mg/dL).

Causes: Acute pancreatitis, vitamin D deficiency, chronic renal insufficiency, burns, malabsorption syndrome, massive blood transfusions.

Assessment Findings: Tetany, convulsions, abdominal and muscle cramps, spasms of larynx and bronchus, circumoral tingling (especially in fingers), confusion, anxiety, moodiness. *ECG changes:* QT interval prolonged, ventricular tachycardia.

Treatment/Nursing Interventions: Calcium gluconate IV, followed by oral calcium supplements as prescribed; serum albumin if condition is due to low serum albumin concentration; monitor for a positive Trousseau's and Chvostek's test; monitor for signs of hypercalcemia and dysrhythmia.

HYPOKALEMIA

. . . .

HYPOMAGNESEMIA

. . . .

Definition: Low concentration of potassium ions in extracellular fluid (serum level lower than 3.5 mEq/L).

Causes: Renal loss (most common—diuretic use), insufficient potassium intake, loss from gastrointestinal tract via nasogastric (NG) tube placement without replacement electrolyte solution, vomiting, diarrhea.

Assessment Findings: Muscle weakness, muscle pain, leg cramps, hyporeflexia, fatigue, hypotension, shallow respirations, dysrhythmias (particularly PVCs), nausea, vomiting, diarrhea, apathy, drowsiness leading to coma, paralytic ileus. *ECG changes:* peaked P waves, flat T wave, depressed ST segment, elevated U waves.

Treatment/Nursing Interventions: Maintain IVs with potassium chloride (KCl) added as prescribed, replace K^+ when excess loss occurs (NG tubes, diarrhea, etc.), observe for adequate urine output.

Special Considerations: Replace no more than 20 mEq of KCl in 1 hour, observe ECG monitor during infusion, dilute KCl in 30–50 mL of IV fluid and administer on an infusion pump.

. . . .

Definition: Deficiency of magnesium due to chronic alcoholism, starvation, malabsorption, or vigorous dieresis (serum level less than 1.3 mg/dL).

Causes: Diet low in magnesium, chronic diarrhea, chemotherapy, pancreatitis, chronic nephritis, diuretic phase of renal failure, toxemia.

Assessment Findings: Jerks, twitches, hyperactive reflexes, tetany, convulsions, coma, tachycardia, ventricular dysrhythmia, hypotension. *ECG changes:* prolonged PR and QT segments.

Treatment/Nursing Interventions: Administrate magnesium sulfate as prescribed, observe for adequate urine output, monitor cardiac rhythm, institute seizure precautions.

Special Considerations: When administering magnesium sulfate, administer intravenously (IV) or intramuscularly (IM) slowly; antidote is calcium gluconate.

. . . .

HYPONATREMIA

- -

MAGNESIUM (Mg) IMBALANCE

- -

POTASSIUM (K⁺) IMBALANCE

PART II

Definition: Low concentration of sodium in extracellular fluid (serum level lower than 135 mEq/L).

Causes: Excessive perspiration, use of diuretics, gastrointestinal losses (severe diarrhea, vomiting, pancreatic and biliary fistula), decreased sodium in diet, burns, excessive IV administration without NaCl, diabetic acidosis, adrenal insufficiency.

Assessment Findings: Weakness, restlessness, delirium, irritability, confusion, hyperpnea, oliguria, increased temperature and pulse, flushed skin, dry mucous membranes, abdominal cramps, convulsions, nausea, anorexia.

Treatment/Nursing Interventions: Administer IV fluids with sodium, maintain accurate intake and output.

Special Considerations: If sodium is lost but fluid is not, the following signs and symptoms will be noted (similar to those of water excess): mental confusion, restlessness, headache, muscle twitching and weakness, oliguria, coma, and convulsions.

. . . .

Normal Serum Value	General Information
1.3–2.1 mEq/L	50% of magnesium is contained in the bones, and the remaining 50% is found in the intracellular compartment.

. . . .

Normal Serum Value	General Information	General Nursing Management
3.5–5.5 mEq/L	• Potassium deficiency and excess are common problems in fluid and electrolyte imbalances. • Major cell cation.	• Observe ECG tracings for changes in T wave, ST segment, or QRS complex. • Measure intake and output accurately. • Draw frequent blood specimens to gauge level. • Observe for signs of metabolic acidosis and alkalosis.

SODIUM (Na) IMBALANCE

. . . .

TONICITY OF IV FLUIDS

. . . .

Normal Serum Value	General Information	General Nursing Management
135–145 mEq/L	• Deficiency and excess are common problems in fluid and electrolyte imbalances.	• Observe skin condition. • Measure intake and output. • Auscultate lung sounds. • Observe specific gravity and color of urine.

	Isotonic	Hypotonic	Hypertonic
Solution	0.9% saline D5W LR	$\frac{1}{2}$ NS $\frac{1}{4}$ NS	D5LR D5$\frac{1}{2}$NS D5NS D10W
Qualities	• Isotonic solutions go where you put them and stay there. • They expand the intravascular space. • Monitor for fluid overload.	• Hypotonic solutions pull water from the intravascular space into the cell. • Less salt and more water. • Cell will swell. • Monitor for cardiovascular collapse.	• Hypertonic solutions greatly expand the intravascular space and draw fluid from intravascular areas. • Cells will shrink.

AFTERLOAD

. . . .

ANEURYSM

. . . .

ANGINA

PART
II

Definition: Resistance to ejection of blood from the ventricle, and the second determinate of stroke volume. The resistance of systemic blood pressure to the left ventricle ejection is called systemic vascular resistance. The resistance of pulmonary blood pressure to the right ventricle is called pulmonary vascular resistance. Afterload has an inverse relationship with stroke volume.

. . . .

Definition: A balloon-like bulge in an artery, resulting from damage or injury to artery walls. They can grow large and rupture, which causes bleeding inside the body, or dissect (split one or more layers of the artery wall), which causes bleeding into and along the layers of the artery wall. Both rupture and dissection are often fatal.

. . . .

Definition: Chest pain as a result of myocardial ischemia related to inadequate myocardial blood and oxygen.
Causes: Obstruction of coronary blood flow from atherosclerosis of the coronary artery, spasms, or any condition that increases myocardial oxygen consumption.
Assessment Findings: Pain, which can develop slowly or quickly; pain described as mild or moderate; pain that is substernal, crushing, or squeezing; pain that may radiate to the arms, back, jaw, shoulders, or neck; pain that can last less than 5 minutes or greater than 20 minutes. Clients may experience dizziness and faintness, dyspnea, digestive disturbances, hypertension, palpations and tachycardia, and sweating.
Treatment/Nursing Interventions: Apply oxygen therapy per order, monitor cardiac signs, assess vital signs, obtain intravenous access, assess pain; institute measures to relieve pain, administer nitroglycerin as ordered, maintain client on bed rest, and obtain a 12-lead electrocardiogram (ECG). Treatment will continue based on client response and healthcare provider orders.
Special Considerations: Various patterns can occur—stable, unstable, intractable or refractory, variant, and preinfarction.

Contra Costa County Library
Brentwood
5/6/2019 4:39:44 PM

- Patron Receipt -
- Renewals -
21901018425946

n Number: 31901054093515
e: NCLEX-RN : flash review /
1ewed
e Date: 5/28/2019 4:39:27 PM

n Number: 31901059199051
e: Lippincott Q & A review for NCLI
1ewed
e Date: 5/28/2019 4:39:34 PM

Contra Costa County Libraries will be
sed on Sunday, April 21st. Items may
renewed at ccclib org or by calling
00-984-4636, menu option 1. Book drops
be open. El Sobrante Library remains
sed for repairs.

ANGINA: TYPES OR PATTERNS OF

. . . .

AORTIC INSUFFICIENCY

. . . .

AORTIC STENOSIS

Type of Angina	Defining Characteristics
Stable Angina (exertional angina)	Predictable and consistent pain that occurs on exertion and is relieved by rest and/or nitroglycerin. Most often has a stable pattern of onset, duration, severity, and relieving factors.
Unstable Angina (preinfarction or crescendo angina)	Symptoms increase in frequency and severity and may not be relieved with rest or nitroglycerin. Increases in occurrence, duration, and severity over time.
Variant Angina (Prinzmetal's angina)	Pain at rest with reversible ST-segment elevations; believed to be caused by coronary spasms. Can occur at rest.
Intractable/Refractory Angina	Chronic, incapacitating pain that is unresponsive to treatment.
Preinfarction Angina	Associated with acute coronary insufficiency. Pain lasts more than 15 minutes. Symptoms are associated with worsening cardiac ischemia. Occurs post myocardial infarction (MI).

· ·

Definition: Incomplete closure of the aortic semilunar valve between the left ventricle and the aorta (regurgitation). Aortic insufficiency results in left ventricular failure, later leading to right ventricular failure.

· ·

Definition: Fusion of the valve flaps between the left ventricle and the aorta. Caused by a congenital abnormality or acquired from atherosclerosis or bacterial endocarditis. Occurs more often in men than in women. Results in pulmonary congestion and decreased cardiac output.

ATRIAL FIBRILLATION

. . . .

BUERGER'S DISEASE (THROMBOANGIITIS OBLITERANS)

. . . .

CARDIAC OUTPUT (CO)

Definition: Rhythm is grossly irregular. Atrial heart rate above 350 beats per minute (can't be counted); ventricular rate will vary with the number of impulses conducted through the AV node. *P wave:* Wavy deflections affecting entire baseline; *PR interval:* Not measurable; *QRS:* Normal (0.10 seconds or less).
Causes: *Risk factors:* Hypertension, diabetes, male gender, congestive heart failure, valvular disease. *Temporary triggers:* Alcohol, cardiac surgery, myocardial infarction (MI), pericarditis, pulmonary embolism.
Assessment Findings: Dependent on ventricular rate. Fatigue, weakness, shortness of breath, distended neck veins, dizziness, anxiety, syncope, palpitations, chest discomfort, hypotension.
Treatment/Nursing Interventions: Antidysrhythmic drugs and anticoagulants (for those at risk of emboli); electric treatment of choice is cardioversion (take anticoagulants for six weeks prior to procedure).
Special Considerations: Clients with atrial fibrillation are at risk for pulmonary embolism and systemic emboli (embolic stroke); careful assessment for these conditions is warranted.

. . . .

Definition: An occlusive disease that causes vasculitis of the small and medium-sized arteries and veins of the extremities. The distal upper and lower limbs are most commonly affected.
Causes: Unknown; strongly associated with tobacco use, familial genetic predisposition, and autoimmune etiologic factors.
Assessment Findings: Claudication (muscle pain caused by inadequate blood supply) of the arch of the foot, intermittent claudication of the lower extremities, aching pain that is more severe at night, sensitivity to cold, pulses diminished in distal extremities; extremities are often cool and red or cyanotic in the dependent position; ulcerations and gangrene may be seen in the digits.
Treatment/Nursing Interventions: No cure; treatment based on symptoms. *Medications:* Vasodilators, antiplatelets, calcium channel blockers.
Special Consideration: Commonly seen in young adult males who smoke.

. . . .

Definition: Refers to the amount of blood pumped by each ventricle during a given period. In a resting adult, this rate is about 5 L/min and varies greatly depending on the metabolic needs of the body. CO is calculated by multiplying the stroke volume by the heart rate.

CATHETERIZATION, CARDIAC

. . . .

CORONARY ANGIOPLASTY, PERCUTANEOUS TRANSLUMINAL (PTCA)

. . . .

CORONARY ARTERY BYPASS GRAFT (CABG)

Definition: A procedure used to diagnose and treat cardiovascular conditions. During the procedure, a long thin tube called a catheter is inserted into an artery or vein in the groin, neck, or arm and threaded through blood vessels to the heart.

. . . .

Definition: A procedure performed to open blocked coronary arteries caused by coronary artery disease (CAD) and to restore arterial blood flow to the heart tissue without open-heart surgery. A catheter is inserted into the coronary artery that is diseased/being treated. This catheter has a tiny balloon at its tip. The balloon is inflated once the catheter has been placed into the narrowed area of the coronary artery. The subsequent inflation of the balloon compresses the fatty tissue in the artery and makes a larger opening inside the artery for improved blood flow. The use of fluoroscopy during the procedure assists the physician in locating blockages as the contrast dye moves through the coronary arteries.

. . . .

Definition: A surgery that improves blood flow to the heart, often in clients diagnosed with severe coronary artery disease (CAD). Open-heart surgery is performed with the use of a cardiopulmonary bypass machine, which allows for full visualization of the heart while maintaining perfusion and oxygenation. During CABG, a healthy artery or vein from the body is connected, or grafted, to the blocked coronary artery. The grafted artery or vein bypasses the blocked portion of the coronary artery. This creates a new passage, and oxygen-rich blood is routed around the blockage to the heart muscle.

CORONARY ARTERY DISEASE (CAD)

• •

**ELECTROCARDIOGRAM (ECG): STEPS
FOR INTERPRETING**

• •

Definition: Also called arteriosclerotic heart disease (ASHD), CAD is a narrowing of the coronary arteries as a result of the accumulation of lipid-containing plaque in the arteries (atherosclerosis).

Causes: Results from inadequate perfusion of the myocardial tissue and decreased myocardial supply, both of which lead to hypertension, angina, dysrhythmia, MI, heart failure, and/or death.

Assessment Findings: Unremarkable findings during asymptomatic periods; chest pains, cough or hemoptysis, excessive fatigue, palpitations, dyspnea, syncope.

Treatment/Nursing Interventions: Instruct client on eliminating risk factors; low-calorie, low-sodium, low-cholesterol, low-fat diet; increased fiber in diet. Surgical treatment may include percutaneous transluminal coronary angioplasty (PTCA), laser angioplasty, atherectomy, vascular stenting, and coronary artery bypass. Medication therapy may include nitrates, calcium channel blockers, cholesterol-lowering medications, and beta-adrenergic blockers (β–blockers).

· ·

Steps: Initially:

1. Determine the heart rate: Count the P waves in a six-second strip to determine the atrial rate, and count the R waves to determine the ventricular rate.

Ask yourself:

2. Is there a QRS complex occurring at regular intervals?

3. Are P waves present for each QRS complex?

Moving on:

4. Measure the PR interval (normal = 0.08–0.20 seconds).

5. Measure the QRS interval (normal = 0.06–0.10 seconds).

6. Identify the T wave and the ST segment.

7. Analyze for any abnormalities.

Essential:

8. Correlate findings with the characteristics of normal sinus rhythm.

9. Identify rhythm.

10. Initiate appropriate treatment modalities.

· ·

ENDOCARDITIS (BACTERIAL, INFECTIVE)

. . . .

HEART FAILURE

. . . .

Definition: An infection of the valves and inner lining, or endocardium, of the heart. Organisms often grow on the endocardium in areas of increased turbulence of blood flow or areas of previous cardiac damage (bacteria can enter from any site of localized infection). Organisms grow on the endocardium, producing vegetation.

Causes: *Risk factors:* History of IV drug abuse, recent invasive procedure, endocarditis, prosthetic valves or valvular disease.

Assessment Findings: Low-grade fever, chills, weakness, malaise, murmur development or change in past murmur, and symptoms of heart failure. *Vascular findings:* Petechia in conjunctiva, lips, buccal mucosa, ankles, and the popliteal and antecubital areas; Osler's nodes on fingertips; and Janeway lesions on the palms and soles of the feet. *Symptoms associated with emboli:* Splenomegaly, upper left quadrant pain, flank pain, hematuria, hemiplegia, decreased level of consciousness, and visual changes.

Treatment/Nursing Interventions: Administer 4 to 6 weeks of antibiotic therapy and bed rest in the presence of a high fever or heart failure. Surgical intervention is required for severe valvular damage.

Special Considerations: Vegetation may invade adjacent valves. Vegetation is fragile and may break off, causing emboli.

. . . .

Definition: A general term used to describe the inadequacy of the heart to pump blood effectively throughout the body. This leads to insufficient perfusion of body tissues with vital nutrients and oxygen. Can be acute or chronic in nature; also referred to as "pump failure."

Causes: Ischemic heart disease, myocardial infarction, cardiomyopathy, valvular heart disease, and hypertension.

Assessment Findings: *Left-sided heart failure* (results in pulmonary congestion due to the inability of the left ventricle to pump blood to the periphery): dyspnea, orthopnea, "wet lungs" cough, fatigue, tachycardia, anxiety, restlessness, and confusion. *Right-sided heart failure* (results in peripheral edema due to the inability of the right ventricle to pump blood out of the lungs): peripheral edema, weight gain, distended neck veins, anorexia, nausea, nocturia, and weakness.

Treatment/Nursing Interventions: Treat the underlying cause, manage hypertension, treat any dysrhythmias, apply oxygen therapy per order, replace potassium as indicated, decrease sodium in the diet, enforce fluid restriction, limit activity, position client in Fowler's or semi-Fowler's position (or seat in an armchair). Medication management includes those that reduce preload and afterload as well as those that improve contractility of the heart: cardiac glycosides, diuretics, aldosterone antagonists, vasodilators, angiotensin-converting enzymes (ACE inhibitors), and beta-blockers.

Special Considerations: Acute pulmonary edema, a medical emergency, can result from left ventricular failure. If not treated, death will occur from suffocation; the client literally drowns in his or her own fluid.

. . . .

HEART SOUNDS

PART II

. . . .

HYPERTENSION: CLASSIFICATION OF

. . . .

	Valve	Location to Listen
Auscultate	Aortic valve (AV)	Right second intercostal space
	Pulmonic valve (PV)	Left second intercostal space
	Tricuspid valve (TV)	Left third and fourth intercostal space
	Mitral valve (MV)	Left midclavicular line
Normal Heart Sounds	S1 (apex)	Closure of the tricuspid and mitral valve (systole): "Lub"
	S2 (base)	Closure of pulmonic and aortic valves (diastole): "Dub"
Abnormal Heart Sounds	S3 (apex)	Rapid ventricular filling: "Ken-tuck-y"
	S4 (tricuspid/mitral)	Increased resistance to ventricular filling: "Ten-nes-see"
	Pericardial friction rub (left sternal border)	Pericardial inflammation: "Grating"
	Other heart sounds	Clicks, snaps, and murmurs

• •

Category	Systolic Blood Pressure (mmHg)		Diastolic Blood Pressure (mmHg)
Normal	<120	and	<80
Prehypertension	120–130	or	80–89
Hypertension Stage I	140–159	or	90–99
Hypertension Stage II	≥160	or	≥100

• •

HYPERTENSION MANAGEMENT

PART II

. . . .

INSUFFICIENCY

. . . .

INTERMITTENT CLAUDICATION

Prehypertension	SBP 120–139, DBP 80–89. Lifestyle modification: weight loss, regular exercise, management of cholesterol levels, reduction of salt intake, and cessation of alcohol and tobacco use.
Hypertension Stage I	SPB 140–159, DBP 90–99. Diuretic therapy (thiazide, loop diuretics, or potassium sparing); may also initiate/consider ACE inhibitor or other antihypertensive medications for blood pressure control.
Hypertension Stage II	SBP 160 or greater, DBP 100 or greater. Continue diuretics; add a second medication, such as a beta-adrenergic blocker, an ACE inhibitor, a calcium channel blocker, or another antihypertensive medication.

SBP = Systolic blood pressure; DBP = Diastolic blood pressure; ACE = Angiotension-converting enzyme.

· ·

Definition: Incomplete closure of a valve due to contraction of chordae tendineae or papillary muscles, or due to calcification and scarring of leaflets.

· ·

Definition: A characteristic leg pain experienced by clients with chronic peripheral arterial disease. Typically, clients can walk only a certain distance before a cramping muscle pain forces them to stop. As the disease progresses, the client can walk only shorter and shorter distances before pain recurs. Eventually, the pain may occur at rest.

MEDICATIONS: ANTIANGINAL

. . . .

MEDICATIONS: ANTIHYPERTENSIVE, I

. . . .

Nitrates
Nitroglycerin
Isosorbide dinitrate (Isordil)
Isosorbide mononitrate (Imdur)
Beta-Blockers
Propranolol HCTZ (Inderal)
Atenolol (Tenormin)
Nadolol (Corgard)
Calcium Channel Blockers
Verapamil (Calan)
Nifedipine HCl (Procardia)
Diltiazem HCl (Cardizem)

Alpha-Adrenergic Blockers
Prazosin (Minipress)
Terazosin (Hytrin)
Phentolamine mesylate (Regitine)
Doxazosin (Cardura)
Combined Alpha Beta-Blockers
Labetalol (Normodyne)
Carvedilol (Coreg)
Beta-Blockers
Metoprolol (Lopressor, Toprol)
Nadolol (Corgard)
Propranolol HCl (Inderal)
Timolol maleate (Blocadren)
Atenolol (Tenormin)
Bisoprolol (Zebeta)

PART II

MEDICATIONS: ANTIHYPERTENSIVE, II

. . . .

MEDICATIONS: DIURETIC

. . . .

Angiotensin-Converting Enzyme (ACE) Inhibitors
Captopril (Capoten)
Enalapril maleate (Vasotec)
Lisinopril (Zestril)
Ramipril (Altace)
Benazepril (Lotensin)
Quinapril (Accupril)
Calcium Channel Blockers
Diltiazem (Cardizem)
Nifedipine (Procardia, Adalat)
Verapamil HCl (Calan, Isoptin)
Nisoldipine (Sular)

Thiazides
Chlorthalidone (Hygroton)
Hydrochlorothiazide (Esidrix, Microzide)
Indapamide (Lozol)
Metolazone (Zaroxolyn)
Loop
Furosemide (Lasix)
Torsemide (Demadex)
Bumetanide (Bumex)
Potassium-Sparing
Spironolactone (Aldactone)
Amiloride (Midamor)

PART II

MEDICATIONS: NITROGLYCERIN ADMINISTRATION, CLIENT EDUCATION FOR

. . . .

MITRAL INSUFFICIENCY

. . . .

MITRAL STENOSIS

1. Bottled sublingual (SL) nitroglycerin must be kept tightly closed and in a dark container.

2. Carry medication at all times (sublingual tablets or translingual spray).

3. Tablets that are fresh will cause a slight tingling/burning sensation when placed under the tongue.

4. Date all medications; discard after 24 months.

5. Prophylactic use: prior to exercise, sexual intercourse, walking, and so on.

6. Take nitroglycerin at the onset of pain and stop all activity.

7. If pain remains after five minutes, call 911 and request Emergency Medical Services (EMS).

8. While waiting for EMS response, if chest pain remains, take another SL tablet or one metered spray.

9. Lie down/remain lying down until EMS arrives.

10. Do not abruptly discontinue.

11. If taking long-acting preparations, schedule an eight-hour nitro-free period each day (at night is recommended).

12. Male clients should not take erectile dysfunction drugs with nitroglycerin.

. . . .

Definition: Leaking/regurgitation of blood back into the left atrium. Mitral insufficiency results from myocardial infarction and chronic rheumatic heart disease. A less common cause is bacterial endocarditis. Men are affected more often than women.

. . . .

Definition: Narrowing of the mitral valve. Most common residual cardiac lesion of rheumatic fever; affects women less than 45 years of age more often than men. Interferes with filling of the left ventricle; produces pulmonary hypertension and right-ventricular failure.

MYOCARDIAL INFARCTION (MI)

. . . .

MYOCARDIAL INFARCTION: CARDIAC ENZYME ELEVATION, POST-MI

. . . .

Definition: Also referred to as coronary occlusion or heart attack. It is considered a total occlusion of a portion of a coronary artery. Following this occlusion, myocardial ischemia, injury, or death occurs.

Causes: *Risk factors:* Atherosclerosis, coronary artery disease (CAD), elevated cholesterol levels, smoking, hypertension, obesity, physical activity, impaired glucose tolerance, and stress.

Assessment Findings: *Pain:* Lasts 30 minutes or longer; crushing substernal; radiates to the jaw, back, and left arm; occurs without cause (often in the morning). Pain is not relieved by rest or nitroglycerin; only relieved by opioid administration. *Other assessment findings:* Diaphoresis, dyspnea, dysrhythmia, feeling fear and anxiety, pallor, cyanosis, and coolness of extremities.

Treatment/Nursing Interventions: *Immediate:* Obtain description of pain, apply nasal cannula oxygen per healthcare provider order, establish IV access, administer nitroglycerin and/or morphine sulfate as ordered, assess vital signs and apply cardiac monitoring, assign bed rest (semi-Fowler's position), obtain 12-lead ECG, administer antidysrhythmic agents and thrombolytic therapy as ordered, monitor laboratory results, administer β-blockers as ordered, and monitor for complications of MI (dysrhythmia, cardiogenic shock, heart failure). Monitor distal pulses, skin temperature, and blood pressure closely after medication administration.

Special Considerations: Not all clients experience the classic symptoms. Women may experience atypical discomfort, shortness of breath, or fatigue, and often present with NSTEMI (non-ST-elevation MI) or T-wave inversion.

Enzyme/Marker	Onset	Peak	Return to Normal
CK-2 (not cardiac specific)	3–6 hours	12–24 hours	3–5 days
CK-MB (recognized indicator of MI by most clinicians)	2–4 hours	12–20 hours	48–72 hours
Myoglobin	1–4 hours (elevates prior to CK-MB)	4–8 hours	24 hours
Cardiac Troponins	As early as 1 hour post-onset	10–24 hours	5–14 days
LDL Total	24 hours	3–6 days	10–14 days
LDH$_1$ (higher LDH$_1$ than LDH$_2$ indicates MI)	12–24 hours	48 hours	10 days
LDH$_2$	12–24 hours	48 hours	10 days

MYOCARDIAL INFARCTION: MONA FOR

. . . .

PACEMAKER, PERMANENT

. . . .

MONA = Immediate treatment of a myocardial infarction (MI)

    M = Morphine

    O = Oxygen

    N = Nitroglycerin

    A = Aspirin or Plavix

Definition	Settings	Pacemaker Spikes
Internal pacemaker with pulse generator implanted in the abdomen or shoulder; can be single or dual chambered. Programmable pacemakers can be reprogrammed by placing a magnetic device over the generator.	Synchronous (demand) pacemaker senses the client's rhythm and paces the heart only when the client's intrinsic rate falls below the set pacemaker rate for stimulating depolarization.	A pacemaker spike (straight vertical line) will be seen on the monitor or electrocardiogram (ECG) strip when a pacing stimulus is delivered to the heart.
	Asynchronous (fixed-rate) pacemaker paces at a fixed rate no matter what the client's intrinsic rhythm is; used when the client is asystolic or severely bradycardic.	Spikes precede the chamber being paced; a spike preceding a P-wave indicates the atrium is being paced; a spike preceding the QRS complex indicates the ventricle is being paced.
	Overriding pacing is used in clients with tachydysrhythmias to suppress the rhythm and permit the sinus node to regain control of the heart.	An atrial spike followed by a P-wave indicates atrial depolarization; a ventricular spike followed by a QRS complex indicates ventricular depolarization; this process is referred to as "pacemaker capture."

PACEMAKER, PERMANENT: CLIENT EDUCATION

. . . .

PACEMAKER, TEMPORARY: INVASIVE EPICARDIAL PACING

. . . .

Instruct client:

- about the pacemaker and programmable rate.
- of the signs of battery failure and when to notify the healthcare provider.
- to report any signs of infection at the insertion site (fever, redness, swelling, and/or drainage).
- to report signs of dizziness, weakness or fatigue, edema of the ankles or legs, chest pain, and/or shortness of breath.
- to carry his or her pacemaker identification card at all times and to obtain and wear a Medic-Alert bracelet.
- how to take a radial pulse daily and to keep a "pulse dairy" of each pulse rate.
- to avoid contact sports.
- to inform all healthcare providers of pacemaker insertion.
- to make airport security aware that he or she has a pacemaker, as it may set off security system.
- that most electronic devices may be used with no interference with pacemaker function.
- to avoid antitheft devices in department stores and transmitter towers.
- to use cell phone on the side opposite the pacemaker.

Type	Definition	Placement	Considerations
Invasive Epicardial Pacing	An electrical power source used outside the body that stimulates and maintains the client's heart rate when the client's intrinsic pacemaker fails to provide a perfusing rhythm (used only in the hospital setting).	Pacing wires applied via transthoracic approach; lead wires are placed on the epicardial surface of the heart after cardiac surgery. Pacemaker wires are brought through the abdomen and capped/covered.	• Insulate the exposed pacer wires with plastic (syringe) or rubber material (rubber glove) when the wires are not attached to the pulse generator. May also cover with nonconductive tape. • Handle pacemaker wires only while wearing rubber gloves to avoid a microshock.

PACEMAKER, TEMPORARY: INVASIVE TRANSVENOUS PACING

. . . .

PACEMAKER, TEMPORARY: NONINVASIVE TRANSVENOUS PACING

. . . .

Type	Definition	Placement	Considerations
Invasive Trans-venous Pacing	An electrical power source used outside the body that stimulates and maintains the client's heart rate when the client's intrinsic pacemaker fails to provide a perfusing rhythm (used only in the hospital setting).	Pacer wires are placed through either the ante-cubital, femoral, jugular, or subclavian vein into the right atrium or right ventricle; this provides direct contact with the endocardium.	• Set pacemaker settings as ordered. • Monitor cardiac rhythm and cardiac status con-tinuously. • Monitor client's vital signs continuously. • Assess pacemaker inser-tion site often. • Restrict client movement to prevent lead wire displacement. • Handle pacemaker wires only while wearing rub-ber gloves to avoid a microshock.

. . . .

Type	Definition	Placement	Considerations
Noninvasive Transvenous Pacing	An electrical power source used outside the body that stimulates and maintains the client's heart rate when the client's intrinsic pacemaker fails to provide a perfusing rhythm (used only in the hospital set-ting).	• Used as a tempo-rary emergency measure in the se-verely bradycardic or asystolic client until a permanent pacemaker can be placed. • Large electrodes/pads are placed on the client's back/posterior (between the spine and left scapula behind the heart; avoid placing over bone) and on the client's chest/anterior (be-tween V2 and V5 positions over the heart; in women place pad under breast tissue).	• Wash skin with soap and water prior to pad/electrode place-ment. • Ensure that the pads/electrodes are in good contact with the skin. • Do not obtain pulse or blood pressure readings on the left side. • Set pacing rate as prescribed; assure pacemaker capture. • Evaluate the client's anxiety and pain level; administer an-algesics as needed.

PAIN ASSESSMENT: PQRST METHOD

· ·

"P" Precipitating Factors	"Q" Quality	"R" Region and Radiation	"S" Symptoms and Signs	"T" Timing and Response to Treatment
• Can occur with or without precipitating factors. • Eating large meals. • Emotional distress. • Physical exertion.	• Burning. • Heaviness. • Increases with movement. • Pressure. • Severe pain. • Smothering.	• Substernal or retrosternal. • Spreads across the chest. • Radiates inside of either or both arms, the back, the jaw, and upper abdomen.	• Apprehension. • Auscultation of crackles and extra heart sounds. • Diaphoresis; cold, clammy skin. • Dyspnea. • Dysrhythmias. • Nausea. • Orthopnea. • Syncope. • Vomiting. • Weakness.	• Sudden onset. • Constant. • Duration greater than 30 minutes. • No relief with nitrates or rest. • Relief with narcotics.

PERICARDITIS

. . . .

PERIPHERAL ARTERIAL DISEASE (PAD)

. . . .

Definition: Inflammation of partial and/or visceral pericardium; acute or chronic condition that may or may not occur with effusion. Fibrosis or accumulation of fluid in the pericardium, which causes compression of cardiac pumping, resulting in decreased cardiac output and increased systemic pulmonic venous pressure.

Causes/Risk Factors: Bacterial, viral, and/or fungal infections, tuberculosis, collagen diseases, uremia, myocardial infarction, and trauma.

Assessment Findings: Sharp pain, which is moderate to severe, located in the area of the pericardium and which may radiate to the right arm, jaw/teeth. Chills, sweating, apprehension, anxiety, fatigue, abdominal pain, shortness of breath, restlessness, tachycardia, elevated temperature, decreased pulse pressure, pulsus paradoxus, pericardial friction rub (hallmark finding). Elevated central venous pressure (CVP), distended neck veins, dependent pitting edema, liver engorgement.

Treatment/Nursing Interventions: Semi-Fowler's position, frequent vital signs with cardiac monitoring, oxygen as ordered. *Medications:* Analgesics, nonsteroidal anti-inflammatory medications, antibiotics, digoxin (Lanoxin), and diuretics if heart failure is noted. *Invasive procedure:* Pericardiocentesis. *Surgical:* Pericardiectomy.

Special Considerations: Monitor for signs of cardiac tamponade, tachycardia, tachypnea, hypotension, pallor, narrow pulse pressure, pulsus paradoxus, or distended neck veins.

· ·

Definition: A chronic disorder in which partial or complete arterial occlusion deprives the lower extremities of oxygen and nutrients. Tissue damage occurs below the level of the occlusion.

Cause: Atherosclerosis.

Assessment Findings: Intermittent claudication, pain at rest with accompanying burning, numbness, and aching in the distal portion of the leg, which awakens the client at night; pain is relieved by placing the limb in the depended position; also, lower back or buttock pain, loss of hair and dry, scaly skin on the lower extremities, thickened toenails, decreased or absent peripheral pulses, elevational pallor and dependent rubor in the lower extremities, signs of arterial ulcer formation, and blood pressure measurements at the thigh, calf, and ankle that are lower than the brachial pressures.

Treatment/Nursing Interventions: Assess pain; monitor the extremities for color, motion, and sensation; check pulses; assess for ulcer formation or signs of gangrene. *Medication therapy:* Antiplatelet agents, antihypertensive agents, and antihyperlipidemic agents. *Procedures to improve arterial blood flow:* Percutaneous transluminal angioplasty, laser-assisted angioplasty, and bypass surgery specific to the area of occlusion.

Special Consideration: Amputation may be necessary.

· ·

PERIPHERAL ARTERIAL DISEASE: CLIENT EDUCATION FOR

. . . .

PHLEBITIS

. . . .

PRELOAD

Instruct client to:

- stop smoking.

- decrease cholesterol and triglyceride intake.

- maintain an optimal body weight.

- adhere to exercise regimen.

- control diabetes and hypertension as directed.

- walk to the point of claudication, stop and rest, and then walk a little farther.

- avoid crossing legs.

- avoid exposure to cold; wear socks as necessary.

- never apply direct heat to the lower extremities.

- inspect skin; report any signs of breakdown to healthcare provider.

. . . .

Definition: When affecting veins on the superficial layer of skin, phlebitis is termed superficial and is not serious; blood clots in the deeper veins are referred to as deep-vein thrombosis. Not serious in its superficial form, though it may herald deep-vein thrombophlebitis, which affects larger blood vessels in the legs; in this form, thrombi or blood clots can break apart and travel to the lungs. This can lead to a life-threatening pulmonary embolism.
Causes: Most common is trauma to the vessel wall caused by an injury to the vein; can also result from prolonged inactivity or a sedentary lifestyle. Other causes: obesity, smoking, pregnancy, certain birth control pills, intravenous drug use, and certain medical conditions like cancer.

. . . .

Definition: Refers to the degree of stretch of the ventricular cardiac muscle fibers at the end of diastole. The end of diastole is the period when the filling volume in the ventricles is the highest and the degree of stretch on the muscle fibers is the greatest. Determined by the volume of blood within the ventricles at the end of diastole; this directly affects stroke volume.

PART II

PULMONARY EDEMA

· ·

RAYNAUD'S PHENOMENON

· ·

Definition: A condition caused by an abnormal accumulation of fluid (blood) in the lung, in both the interstitial and alveolar spaces. Pulmonary edema is a result of severe impairment of the left side of the heart to maintain cardiac output, leading to engorgement of the pulmonary bed.

Causes: *Risk factors:* Inhaled toxins, severe hypoxia, pneumonia, cardiac myopathy, heart failure, and overhydration.

Assessment Findings: *Initial findings:* Frothy-pink (blood-tinged) sputum (classic sign), restlessness, anxiousness, sense of breathlessness and suffocation, ashen skin, weakened and thready pulse, distended neck veins. *Late findings:* Confusion, stupor, breathing that is rapid, noisy, and moist-sounding; oxygen saturation readings decrease drastically.

Treatment/Nursing Interventions: Oxygen therapy via a face mask (mechanical ventilation may be required), obtain IV access, administer IV morphine, IV push or a continuous infusion of Lasix/Furosemide, and an IV infusion of a vasodilator (nitroglycerin or nitroprusside [Nipride]) per physician order, position client in a high Fowler's position, insert a Foley catheter, monitor vital signs and urine output, and provide emotional support.

Special Consideration: Pulmonary edema is a medical emergency and requires prompt recognition and treatment.

• •

Definition: An episodic vasospastic disorder of small cutaneous arteries, most frequently involving the fingers and toes. The vasospasms result from an exaggerated response to the sympathetic nervous stimulation.

Causes: *Contributing factors:* Occupationally related trauma and pressure to the fingertips (pianists, typists, and those who handle vibrating equipment). Exposure to stress, cold, caffeine, and tobacco.

Assessment Findings: Vasospasm-induced color changes of the fingers, ears, nose, and toes (white, blue, and red). Complaints of coldness, numbness, throbbing, aching pain; tingling and swelling of the affected area during an attack. After frequent, prolonged attacks, skin will thicken and nails will become brittle.

Treatment/Nursing Interventions: *Extensive client teaching:* Avoidance of temperature extremes (cold), tobacco and caffeine use, and stress. *Medications:* Calcium channel blockers (Nifedipine/Procardia; Diltiazem/Cardizem).

Special Consideration: Commonly seen in young adult women between the ages of 15 and 40.

• •

SHOCK STATES

PART II

Shock State	Signs and Symptoms	Nursing Intervention/Treatment
Hypovolemic	Pallor, cool, clammy skin; ↓ BP; rapid, thready pulse; shallow respirations, ↓ UO; changes in LOC	Oxygen, rapid infusion of fluid volume (blood, crystalloids). Correct the cause (e.g., bleeding, GI losses).
Cardiogenic	Pallor, cool, clammy skin; ↓ BP, rapid, thready pulse; tachypnea; crackles; ronchi; ↓ UO; ↓ BS; changes in LOC	Oxygen, hemodynamic monitoring, nitrates, inotropes, diuretics. Restore blood flow.
Anaphylactic	Cool, pale skin; ↓ BP; ↑ pulse; chest pains; swelling of the lips and/or tongue, larynx, epiglottis; wheezing; stridor; skin rash; anxiety	Oxygen, fluid resuscitation, antihistamines, epinephrine, bronchodilators, corticosteroids. Identify and remove cause.
Neurogenic	Pale, warm, dry skin; ↓ BP; ↓ pulse	Oxygen, cautious use of fluid resuscitation, vasopressors, atropine. Treatment dependent on cause (e.g., spinal cord injury).
Septic	Flushed, pale, cyanotic skin; BP normal, ↓ BP; full, bounding pulse; rapid, weak, thready, shallow respirations; changes in LOC	Oxygen, hemodynamic monitoring, aggressive fluid resuscitation, antibiotics (cultures first, e.g., blood, urine, wound), vasopressors, inotropes.

↓ = Decreased; ↑ = Increased; BP = Blood pressure; BS = Bowel sounds; GI = Gastrointestinal; LOC = Level of consciousness; UO = Urine output.

SINUS BRADYCARDIA

. . . .

SINUS RHYTHM, NORMAL

. . . .

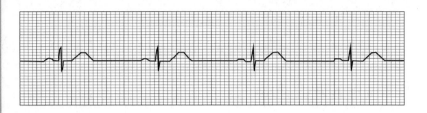

Definition: Heart rate below 60 beats per minute; P wave: one for every QRS complex; PR interval: normal (0.12–0.20 seconds); QRS complex: normal (0.10 seconds or less).

Causes: Hypoxia, myocardial infarction (inferior wall), suctioning, vomiting, valsalva maneuvers, beta-adrenergic blocking agents, calcium channel blockers, digitalis.

Assessment Findings: Syncope, dizziness and weakness, confusion, hypotension, diaphoresis, shortness of breath, and angina pain.

Treatment/Nursing Interventions: Oxygen therapy, external pacemaker, atropine intravenously (IV).

Special Considerations: Well-conditioned athletes have a hypereffective heart, thus tolerating bradycardia well.

· ·

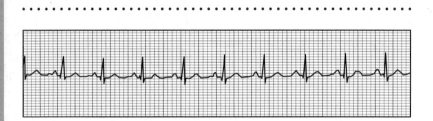

Definition: Heart rate below 60–80 beats per minute; rhythm is regular; P wave: one for every QRS complex; PR interval: normal (0.12–0.20 seconds); QRS complex: normal (0.10 seconds or less).

· ·

SINUS TACHYCARDIA

. . . .

STENOSIS

. . . .

STROKE VOLUME (SV)

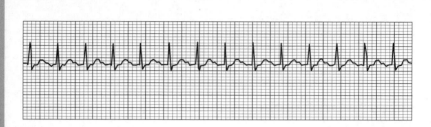

Definition: Heart rate between 100 and 180 beats per minute; P wave: one for every QRS complex; PR interval: normal (0.12–0.20 seconds); QRS complex: normal (0.10 seconds or less).

Causes: Excitement, exertion, fever, infection, septic shock, hypoxia, hypovolemia, hypotension, heart failure, pain, anxiety, anemia, smoking, alcohol, caffeine, medications that increase sympathetic tone, medications that decrease parasympathetic tone, myocardial ischemia, and myocardial infarction.

Assessment Findings: Fatigue, weakness, restlessness, anxiety, shortness of breath, orthopnea, neck vein distension, decreased oxygen saturation, and hypotension.

Treatment/Nursing Interventions: Treat the underlying cause. Initiate oxygen and medication therapy as directed.

Special Considerations: Sinus tachycardia in healthy individuals is usually benign and does not require aggressive treatment. The underlying cause must be treated.

· ·

Definition: Narrowing of valvular opening due to adherence, thickening, and rigidity of valve cusp. This narrowing prevents the valve from opening fully, which obstructs blood flow from the heart into the aorta and onward to the rest of the body. When the aortic valve is obstructed, the heart needs to work harder to pump blood to the body, which eventually can weaken the heart and limits the amount of blood it can pump, leading to symptoms, such as fatigue and dizziness. In its severe form, surgery is required to replace the valve. Left untreated, it can lead to serious heart problems.

· ·

Definition: Amount of blood ejected from the ventricle per heartbeat. The average resting stroke volume is about 70 mL, and the heart rate is 60–80 bpm. Cardiac output can be affected by changes in either stroke volume or heart rate.

VALVULAR DEFECTS: COMPARISON OF SYMPTOMATOLOGY OF, I

. . . .

VALVULAR DEFECTS: COMPARISON OF SYMPTOMATOLOGY OF, II

. . . .

Assessment Subjective Data	Mitral Stenosis	Mitral Insufficiency	Aortic Stenosis	Aortic Insufficiency
Fatigue	x	x	x	x
Shortness of Breath	x		x	x
Orthopnea	x		x	x
Proximal Nocturnal Dyspnea		x	x	x
Cough	x	x		
Dyspnea of Exertion		x	x	x
Palpitations		x	x	x
Syncope of Exertion			x	
Angina			x	
Weight Loss		x		

Assessment Objective Data	Mitral Stenosis	Mitral Insufficiency	Aortic Stenosis	Aortic Insufficiency
Blood Pressure: Low Normal	x	x		
Blood Pressure: Normal or Elevated			x	x
Pulse: Weak, Irregular	x	x		
Pulse: Rapid				x
Respirations: Increased, Shallow	x	x		
Dyspnea of Exertion	x			
Cyanosis	x			
Jugular Vein Distention	x			
Enlarged Liver	x		x	
Murmur	x	x	x	x

VENOUS THROMBOSIS (THROMBOPHLEBITIS)

. . . .

VENTRICULAR CONTRACTIONS/COMPLEXES, PREMATURE (PVCs)

. . . .

Definition: The most common disorder of the veins; the formation of a thrombosis (clot) in association with inflammation of the vein. Can be superficial or a deep-vein thrombosis (DVT).

Causes: *Risk factors (Virchow's triad): Venous stasis:* Surgery (hip, pelvic, and orthopedic surgery); pregnancy, obesity; prolonged immobility; heart disease. *Endothelial damage:* IV fluid and drug use; abdominal and pelvic surgery; history of DVT; fractures and dislocations (leg, hip, pelvis). *Hypercoagulability:* Malignancies, dehydration; blood dyscrasias; oral contraceptives.

Assessment Findings: Superficial thrombophlebitis: firm, palpable, cord-like vein; tender to touch; surrounding area warm and reddened. DVT: Area around vein is tender to touch, reddened, and warm; extremity pain and edema; temperature above 100.4°F; Homan's sign may be present but is an unreliable indicator.

Treatment/Nursing Interventions: Bed rest; elevate extremity; anticoagulation, anti-inflammatory, and fibrinolytic medications; warm, moist packs; elastic support stocking on unaffected extremity during periods of bed rest; surgical interventions: venous thrombectomy, umbrella filter in the vena cava.

Special Consideration: DVT is associated with a high risk for pulmonary emboli, chronic venous insufficiency, and venous stasis ulcers.

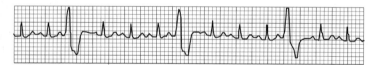

Definition: An impulse that starts in the ventricle and is conducted through the ventricles before the next normal sinus impulse.

Causes: Cardiac ischemia or infarction, heart failure, tachycardia, digitalis toxicity, hypoxia, acidosis, or electrolyte imbalances, especially hypokalemia. Underlying rhythm can be regular or irregular. P wave is not usually visible and is often hidden in the PVC; PR interval is not measurable; QRS complex is wide and distorted.

Assessment Findings: Can be benign in those with no underlying heart disease. In heart disease, depending on frequency, can reduce cardiac output and precipitate angina and heart failure.

Treatment/Nursing Interventions: Treatment is based on the cause of the PVC (e.g., oxygen therapy for hypoxia, electrolyte replacement). Medication therapy may consist of beta-blockers, procainamide, amiodarone, or lidocaine.

Special Considerations: PVCs can occur in healthy people with intake of caffeine, nicotine, or alcohol. PVCs can be called as follows: bigeminy—every other complex is a PVC; trigeminy—every third complex is a PVC; and quadrigeminy—every fourth complex is a PVC.

VENTRICULAR FIBRILLATION (VF)

. . . .

VENTRICULAR TACHYCARDIA (VT)

. . . .

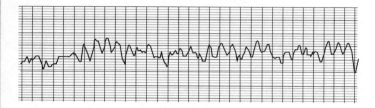

Definition: A severe derangement of the heart rhythm characterized on the ECG by irregular undulations of varying shapes and amplitude. HR is not measurable. Rhythm is irregular and chaotic. The P wave is not visible, and the PR interval and QRS interval are not measurable.

Causes: Acute myocardial infarction, myocardial ischemia, CAD, cardiomyopathy, electrical shock, hyperkalemia, hypoxia, acidosis, and drug toxicity.

Assessment Findings: Unresponsiveness, pulselessness, and apneic state.

Treatment/Nursing Interventions: Immediate CPR and advanced cardiac life support (ACLS) measures, with the use of defibrillation and definitive medication therapy.

Special Consideration: Mechanically, the ventricle is simply quivering and not effectively contracting; consequently, no cardiac output occurs.

• •

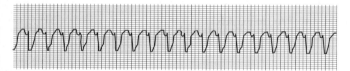

Definition: Three or more PVCs in a row. It occurs when there is an ectopic focus, or when foci fire repetitively and the ventricle takes control as the pacemaker. Ventricular rate is 150–250 bpm. Rhythm is regular or irregular; P waves occur independently of the QRS complex; the P wave can be buried in the QRS complex, and the PR interval is not measurable. The QRS complex is distorted in appearance, with duration greater than 0.12 seconds. It can be stable (with a pulse) or unstable (without a pulse).

Causes: Associated with myocardial infarction, CAD, significant electrolyte imbalances, cardiomyopathy, mitral valve prolapse, digitalis toxicity, and central venous disorders.

Assessment Findings: Hypotension, pulmonary edema, decreased cerebral blood flow, and cardiopulmonary arrest.

Treatment/Nursing Interventions: *Stable:* Beta-blockers, lidocaine, amiodarone, procainamide, or sotalol. *Unstable:* Cardiopulmonary resuscitation (CPR) with rapid defibrillation are first-line treatments, followed by epinephrine if defibrillation is unsuccessful.

Special Consideration: Occurrence without a pulse is life-threatening.

• •

PART
II

ADDISON'S CRISIS

. . . .

ADDISON'S DISEASE

. . . .

CHVOSTEK'S SIGN

Definition: A life-threatening disorder caused by adrenal hormone insufficiency. Crisis is precipitated by infection, trauma, stress, or surgery. Death may occur from shock, vascular collapse, or hyperkalemia.

Causes: Severe physical shock (e.g., a car accident); severe infection (e.g., flu with a high temperature); severe dehydration (e.g., stomach bug with vomiting).

Assessment Findings: Extreme weakness; mental confusion; extreme drowsiness, in advanced cases slipping toward a coma; pronounced dizziness; nausea and/or vomiting; severe headache; abnormal heart rate (bradycardia or tachycardia); abnormally low blood pressure; feeling extremely cold; possibly a fever or abdominal tenderness.

· ·

Definition: Autoimmunity-induced condition resulting in a decrease in secretion of the adrenal cortex hormones; decreased physiologic response to stress, vascular insufficiency, and hypoglycemia; can cause an alteration in adrenal androgen secretion necessary for secondary sex characteristics.

Causes: Occurs after bilateral adrenalectomy or abrupt withdrawal from long-term corticosteroid therapy; adrenal crisis may be precipitated by client's failure to take medications, AIDS, septicemia, tuberculosis, or increased emotional stress without appropriate hormone replacement.

Assessment Findings: Fatigue, weakness, weight loss, gastrointestinal (GI) disturbances, hypoglycemia, postural hypotension, hyponatremia, hyperkalemia, bronze pigmentation of the skin, and Addisonian crisis.

Treatment/Nursing Interventions: Focus on replacement of adrenal hormones and safely administering steroid replacement; frequently evaluate vital signs, assess sodium and water retention, evaluate serum potassium levels, and keep client immobilized and quiet. Administer steroid preparations with food or antacid, evaluate for edema and fluid retention, assess serum sodium and potassium levels, check daily weight, increase intake of protein and carbohydrates, monitor for cushingoid symptoms, and evaluate for hypoglycemia.

· ·

Definition: An abnormal spasm of the facial muscles, elicited by light taps on the cheek to stimulate the facial nerves in clients who are hypocalcemic. It is a sign of tetany. Checking for this sign is especially important after thyroid or parathyroid surgery.

PART II

CUSHING'S DISEASE

· ·

DIABETES INSIPIDUS

· ·

DIABETES MELLITUS

Definition: Condition resulting from excess levels of adrenal cortex hormones and, to a lesser extent, androgen and aldosterone.

Causes: More common in women (20–40 years old); pituitary hypersecretion, a benign pituitary tumor, iatrogenic (most often a result of long-term steroid therapy).

Assessment Findings: Emotional lability and irritability; moon face; deposit of fat on the back; thin skin, purple striae; truncal obesity with thin extremities; petechiae and bruises; persistent hyperglycemia; GI distress from increased acid production; osteoporosis; increased risk of infection; edema; potassium depletion; hypertension; amenorrhea (females); hirsutism (females); gynecomastia (males); impotence or decreased libido.

Treatment/Nursing Interventions: Manage hormone imbalance directed at restricting sodium and water intake, monitor fluid and electrolyte levels, evaluate for hyperglycemia and GI disturbances, and prevent infection. Identify complications, including excess sodium and water retention, potassium depletion, thromboembolic problems, and fractures.

• •

Definition: The hyposecretion of antidiuretic hormone from the posterior pituitary gland, resulting in failure of tubular reabsorption of water in the kidneys and diuresis.

• •

Definition: A complex, multisystem disease characterized by the absence of, or a severe decrease in, the secretion or utilization of insulin. Classified as either type 1 (absolute lack of insulin secretion) or type 2 (combination of insulin resistance and inadequate insulin secretion to compensate). Clinical manifestations of both type 1 and type 2 include polyphagia, polydipsia, polyuria, fatigue, and increased frequency of infections.

DIABETES, TYPE 1

. . . .

DIABETES, TYPE 2

. . . .

Description:

- Absolute lack of insulin secretion.

- Previously known as juvenile diabetes or insulin-dependent diabetes mellitus.

- Absence of insulin production; client is dependent on insulin to prevent ketoacidosis and maintain life.

- Onset is frequently in childhood; most often diagnosed before the age of 18 years. Most common age range is 10 to 15 years.

- Familial tendencies in transmission.

- Lifelong disorder.

Clinical Manifestations: Weight loss, excessive thirst, bed-wetting, blurred vision, and abdominal pain.

• •

Description:

- Combination of insulin resistance and inadequate insulin secretion to compensate.

- Insulin deficiency caused by defects in insulin production or excessive demands for insulin; client is not dependent on insulin.

- Ketoacidosis not a concern.

- Onset is predominately in adulthood, generally after the age of 40 years, but it may occur at any age; previously called adult onset diabetes mellitus (AODM) or non-insulin-dependent diabetes.

- Associated with obesity; obese clients require more insulin.

- Blood sugar is often controlled by diet and oral hypoglycemics, but during episodes of increased stress insulin injections may be required.

Clinical Manifestations:

- Clients often asymptomatic for the first 5–10 years.

- Weight gain.

- Visual disturbances; fatigue and malaise.

- Recurrent vaginal yeast or monilia infections (frequently initial symptom in women).

• •

DIABETIC KETOACIDOSIS (DKA)

· ·

DKA AND HHNS, DIFFERENCES BETWEEN

· ·

HYPERGLYCEMIA

Definition: A life-threatening complication of diabetes mellitus that develops when a severe insulin deficiency occurs. Hyperglycemia progresses to this state over a period of several hours to several days. Acidosis occurs in clients with type 1 diabetes mellitus, persons with undiagnosed diabetes, and persons who stop prescribed treatment for diabetes.

· ·

	DKA	HHNS
Onset/Age	Sudden/All ages, with increased incident in children	Gradual/Adult (usually seen in older adults with chronic illness)
Precipitating Factors	Infection, other stressors, inadequate insulin dose	Infection, other stressors, poor fluid intake
Manifestations	• Ketosis: Kussmaul's respirations, fruity breath, nausea, abdominal pain • Dehydration or electrolyte loss: polyuria, polydipsia, weight loss, dry skin, sunken eyes, soft eyeballs, lethargy, coma	• Altered central nervous system function with neurologic symptoms • Dehydration or electrolyte loss: same as DKA

· ·

Definition: Elevated blood glucose level greater than 250 mg/dL.
Clinical Findings: High blood glucose levels, high levels of sugar in the urine, frequent urination, increased thirst.

HYPERGLYCEMIC HYPEROSMOLAR NONKETOTIC SYNDROME (HHNS)

. . . .

HYPERPITUITARISM

. . . .

HYPERTHYROIDISM/GRAVES' DISEASE

Definition: Extreme hyperglycemia without acidosis. A complication of type 2 diabetes mellitus that may result in dehydration or vascular collapse but does not include the acidosis component of diabetic ketoacidosis. Onset is usually slow, taking from hours to days.

. . . .

Definition: Hypersecretion of growth hormone by the anterior pituitary gland; leads to conditions such as acromegaly and Cushing's disease.
Causes: Primarily by pituitary tumors.
Assessment Findings: Large hands and feet, thickening and protrusion of the jaw, arthritic changes and joint pain, visual disturbances, diaphoresis, oily and rough skin, organomegaly, hypertension, dysphagia, and deepening of the voice.
Treatment/Nursing Interventions: Provide emotional support and encouragement to the client and family to express feelings related to disturbed body image, provide frequent skin care, provide pharmacological and non-pharmacological interventions for joint pain, prepare the client for radiation of pituitary gland if indicated, and prepare the client for hypophysectomy if planned.

. . . .

Definition: An immune system disorder that results in the overproduction of thyroid hormones.
Causes: More prevalent in women and older adults; peak incidence in third and fourth decade of life; possibly an autoimmune condition.
Assessment Findings: Because thyroid hormones affect several body systems, signs and/or symptoms (s/s) can be wide-ranging; they include anxiety; irritability; difficulty sleeping; fatigue; rapid or irregular heartbeat; fine tremor of hands or fingers; increase in perspiration or warm, moist skin; sensitivity to heat; weight loss, despite normal eating habits; goiter; change in menstrual cycles; erectile dysfunction or reduced libido; frequent bowel movements or diarrhea; bulging eyes; and thick, red skin usually on the shins or tops of the feet.
Treatment/Nursing Interventions: Thyroidectomy; reduction of thyroid tissue; irradiation of thyroid gland, eventually resulting in hypothyroid state; decreased thyroid synthesis and release. Other interventions involve decreasing the effects of excess thyroid hormone, preventing complications of thyroid storm, and protecting the eyes.

PART II

HYPOGLYCEMIA

· ·

HYPOPITUITARISM

· ·

HYPOTHYROIDISM

Definition: Decreased blood glucose level, lower than 70 mg/dL, which results from too much insulin, not enough food, or excess activity.

Clinical Findings:

- *Mild:* Hunger, nervousness, palpitations, sweating, tachycardia, tremor.
- *Moderate:* Confusion, drowsiness, double vision, headache, impaired coordination, inability to concentrate, irrational or combative behavior, slurred speech, numbness of tongue and lips.
- *Severe:* Difficulty arousing, seizures, loss of consciousness.

• •

Definition: Hyposecretion of one or more of the pituitary hormones caused by tumors, trauma, encephalitis, autoimmunity, or stroke. Hormones most often affected are growth hormone (GH) and gonadotropic hormones (luteinizing hormone, follicle-stimulating hormone); thyroid-stimulating hormone (TSH), adrenocorticotropic hormone (ACTH), or antidiuretic hormone (ADH) may be involved.

Assessment Findings: Mild to moderate obesity (GH, TSH), reduced cardiac output (GH, ADH), infertility, sexual dysfunction (gonadotropins, ACTH), fatigue, low blood pressure (TSH, ADH, ACTH, GH), tumors of the pituitary also may cause headaches and visual defects (pituitary is located near the optic nerve).

Treatment/Nursing Interventions: Provide emotional support to the client/family; encourage the client/family to express feelings related to disturbed body image or sexual dysfunction; client may need hormone replacement for the specific deficient hormones; client education is needed regarding the signs and symptoms of hypofunction and hyperfunction related to insufficient or excess hormone replacement.

• •

Definition: Condition characterized by a slow deterioration of thyroid function; occurs primarily in older adults and five times more frequently in women (ages 30–60) than in men. Myxedema coma is a life-threatening form.

Causes: Hyposecretion of thyroid hormones T_3 and T_4.

Assessment Findings: *Early:* Extreme fatigue, menstrual disturbances, brittle nails, hair loss, dry skin, anorexia, intolerance to cold, apathy, constipation. *Late:* Subnormal temperature, bradycardia, congestive heart failure, hypotension, thickened skin, weight gain and edema, alterations in level of consciousness.

Treatment/Nursing Interventions: Assist client to return to hormone balance: thyroid replacement; provide a warm environment; prevent and treat constipation; assess client's response to therapy (decreased body weight, intake and output balance, reduction in visible edema, increased energy level); evaluate cardiovascular response to medications. Assist the client to understand implications of disease and requirements for health maintenance.

INSULIN, TYPES OF: INTERMEDIATE-ACTING AND LONG-ACTING

. . . .

INSULIN, TYPES OF: RAPID-ACTING AND SHORT-ACTING

. . . .

Type/Description	Onset	Peak	Duration
Intermediate-Acting Insulin: NPH/Lente (Humulin N, Novolin N, ReliOn) • Never give IV. • May be mixed with regular insulin.	2–4 hours	4–10 hours	10–16 hours
Long-Acting Insulin: Glargine (Lantus), detemir (Levemir) • Glargine has a low pH (4). • Cannot be mixed with other insulins. • Usually given once a day at bedtime, but can be administered during the day.	1–2 hours	No pronounced peak	24+ hours

Type/Description	Onset	Peak	Duration
Rapid-Acting Insulin: Lispro (Humalog), aspart (NovoLog), glulisine (Apidra) • Should be used in combination with long-acting insulin. • Because of quick onset and action, client must eat immediately.	15 minutes	60–90 minutes	3–4 hours
Short-Acting Insulin: Regular (Humulin R, Novolin R, ReliOn N) • Given 20–30 minutes before meals. • May be given alone or in combination with longer-acting insulins. • Given for sliding-scale coverage. • May mix regular insulin with other insulins. • Only regular insulin may be given IV.	$\frac{1}{2}$–1 hour	2–3 hours	3–6 hours

MYXEDEMA

· ·

SOMOGYI PHENOMENON

· ·

THYROID STORM

· ·

TROUSSEAU'S SIGN

Definition: The most severe form of hypothyroidism characterized by swelling of the hands, face, feet, and periorbital tissues. At this stage, the disease may lead to coma and death.

· ·

Definition: A rebound phenomenon that occurs in clients with type 1 diabetes mellitus. Normal or evaluated blood glucose levels are present at bedtime; hypoglycemia occurs at about 2 to 3 a.m. Counterregulatory hormones, produced to prevent further hypoglycemia, result in hyperglycemia (evident in the pre-breakfast blood glucose level). Treatment includes decreasing the evening (pre-dinner or bedtime) dose of intermediate-acting insulin or increasing the bedtime snack.

· ·

Definition: An acute, potentially fatal exacerbation of hyperthyroidism that may result from manipulation of the thyroid gland during surgery, severe infection, or stress. Antithyroid medications, β-blockers (beta-blockers), glucocorticoids, and iodides may be administered before thyroid surgery to prevent its occurrence.

· ·

Definition: A sign of hypocalcemia. Carpel spasm can be elicited by compressing the brachial artery with a blood pressure cuff for 3 minutes.

CATARACTS

. . . .

EAR DROPS, ADMINISTRATION OF

. . . .

EYEDROPS, ADMINISTRATION OF

Definition: Condition characterized by opacity of the lens. Diagnostic tests include ophthalmoscope and slip-lamp biomicroscope. Surgical removal is done when vision impairment interferes with daily activities.
Causes: Advanced age; trauma, toxic substances, or systemic diseases; or may be congenital.
Assessment Findings: *Early signs:* Blurred vision, decreased color perception. *Late signs:* Diplopia; reduced visual acuity, progressing to blindness; clouded pupil, progressing to a milky-white appearance.
Treatment/Nursing Interventions: Postoperative care: teach proper eye medication instillation to client or family member. Postoperative teaching includes: Client should not rub or apply pressure to the operative eye; shaded glasses should be worn during waking hours and an eyelid cover during sleeping hours; take stool softeners to avoiding straining; no lifting of 15 pounds or more, bending, coughing, or any other activity that may increase intraocular pressure; avoid lying on operative side; keep water out of eye while showering; report pain or changes in vital signs.

. . . .

Note: Remember to pull the ear up and back.

1. Position the client on the side of the unaffected ear (or tilt the head). Pull the pinna up and back.

2. Direct the ear drops toward the ear canal (this is done to avoid hitting the tympanic membrane, which would cause pain) and instill the correct number of drops.

3. Release the pinna.

4. Instruct the client to remain in the tilted head position for 2 to 3 minutes to allow solution to run completely in the ear.

5. Instruct the client to resume a normal head position, and dry any solution from around the outside of the ear.

. . . .

1. Retract the client's lower eyelid gently.

2. Request that the client look up at the ceiling to diminish the corneal reflex.

3. Instill the eyedrops into the inner corner of the eye (conjunctival sac).

4. Gently release the client's lid.

Note: Never let the drop(s) fall directly on the pupil.

GLAUCOMA

. . . .

HEARING LOSS, TYPES OF

. . . .

HYPEROPIA

Definition: A group of ocular diseases resulting in increased intraocular pressure. Increased pressure results from inadequate drainage of aqueous humor from the canal of Schlemm or overproduction of the aqueous humor. The condition damages the optic nerve and can result in blindness. Cannot be cured but can be treated successfully with medications and surgery.
Causes: Family history, history of diabetes, increased incident in the elderly, certain medications (antihistamines, anticholinergics).
Assessment Findings: *Early signs:* Increased intraocular pressure, greater than 22 mmHg; decreased accommodation or ability to focus. *Late signs:* Loss of peripheral vision; seeing halos around light; decreased visual acuity not correctable with glasses; headache or eye pain that may be so severe as to cause nausea and vomiting.
Treatment/Nursing Interventions: Administer eyedrops as ordered (Pilocarpine most commonly utilized); teach client about proper eyedrop administration, safety measures, and avoiding activities that increase intraocular pressure.
Special Considerations: Vision that is lost cannot be restored; eyedrops will be required for life. Instruct client that after Pilocarpine administration vision may be blurred for 1 to 2 hours, and adaptation to dark environments will be difficult because of papillary constriction (desired effects of medication).

Conductive Hearing Loss	Hearing loss in which sound does not travel well to the sound organs of the inner ear. The volume of sound is less, but the sound remains clear. If voice volume is raised, hearing is normal. Usually results from cerumen (wax) impaction or middle ear disorders. Treated successfully with hearing aids.
Sensorineural Hearing Loss	A form of hearing loss in which sound passes properly through the outer and middle ear but is distorted by a defect in the inner ear. Involves perceptual loss, usually progressive and bilateral. Damage to the eighth cranial nerve. Causes include infections, ototoxic drugs, trauma, neuromas, noise, aging process.

Definition: Farsightedness; rays coming from an object converge to a point behind the retina. Vision beyond 20 feet is normal, but near vision is poor. Condition corrected by a convex lens.

MACULAR DEGENERATION

. . . .

MYDRIASIS

. . . .

Definition: A blurred central vision caused by progressive degeneration of the center of the retina. The condition may be atrophic or age-related, and may be dry or exudative (wet).

. . . .

Definition: A dilated pupil that occurs because of blockage of the muscarinic receptors of the sphincter muscles or by stimulation of the alpha receptors of the dilator muscles. Enlarged pupils occur with stimulation of the sympathetic nervous system, use of dilating drops, acute glaucoma, or past or recent surgery.

. . . .

MYOPIA

. . . .

RETINAL DETACHMENT

. . . .

Definition: Nearsightedness; rays coming from an object are focused in the front of the retina. Near vision is normal, but distant vision is altered. A biconcave lens is used for correction.

· ·

Definition: A hole or tear in, or separation of the sensory retina from, the pigmented epithelium. Occurs when the layers of the retina separate because of the accumulation of fluid between them, or when both retinal layers elevate away from the choroid as a result of a tumor. Partial detachment becomes complete when untreated. When detachment becomes complete, blindness occurs.
Causes: Blunt-trauma astigmatism.
Assessment Findings: Flashes of light; floaters or black spots (signs of bleeding), increasing blurred vision, loss of a portion of the visual field, painless loss of central or peripheral vision.
Treatment/Nursing Interventions: Client may be placed on bed rest; eye patch placed over affected eye; administer medication as ordered to inhibit accommodation and constriction; cycloplegics (mydriatic and homatropine) are administered to dilate the pupil prior to surgery; administer pain medication postoperatively as ordered (Tylenol, Demerol, Oxycodone); if gas bubble used (inserted in vitreous), position client so bubble can rise against area to be reattached.
Special Considerations: Resealing is done by surgery: cryotherapy (freezing), photocoagulation (laser), diathermy (heat), or scleral buckling (most common).

· ·

ASCITES

....

BOWEL (OR INTESTINAL) OBSTRUCTION

....

CHOLECYSTITIS

Definition: Accumulation of fluid (usually serous fluid, which is a pale yellow and clear fluid) in the abdominal/peritoneal cavity. Ascitic fluid can have many sources, such as liver disease, cancers, congestive heart failure, or kidney failure. The most common cause is advanced liver disease.

. . . .

Definition: Obstruction that occurs when the small or large intestine is partly or completely blocked, which prevents food, fluids, and gas from moving through the intestines normally. Fluid, gas, and intestinal contents accumulate proximal to the obstruction. This causes distention proximal to the obstruction and bowel collapse distal to the obstruction.
Causes: Can be mechanical or intestinal/vascular. Mechanical causes include strangulated hernia, intussusceptions, volvulus, tumors, adhesions, vascular obstruction.
Assessment Findings: Vomiting, abdominal distention; initially bowel sounds may be hyperactive proximal to the obstruction and decreased or absent distal to the obstruction; eventually all bowel sounds will be absent; paralytic ileus or adynamic ileus, colicky abdominal pain, fluid and electrolyte imbalance (dehydration).
Treatment/Nursing Interventions: Medical and vascular obstruction are generally treated surgically; ileostomy or colostomy may be necessary; conservative treatment includes nasogastric (NG) suctioning and decompression; fluid and electrolyte replacement. If intussusception is noted: hydrostatic reduction by water-soluble contrast, air or barium enema.

. . . .

Definition: An inflammation of the gallbladder, which is frequently associated with stones; this condition may be acute or chronic.
Causes: Associated with stones; *Escherichia coli* is a common bacterium involved; may also be associated with neoplasms, anesthesia, or adhesions.
Assessment Findings: Nausea and vomiting, indigestion, belching, flatulence, epigastric pain that radiates to the scapula 2 to 4 hours after eating fatty foods and may persist for 4 to 6 hours; pain localized in the right upper quadrant; guarding, rigidity, and rebound tenderness; Murphy's sign, elevated temperature, tachycardia, signs of dehydration. If biliary obstruction is present: jaundice, dark orange and foamy urine, steatorrhea and clay-colored feces, pruritus.
Treatment/Nursing Interventions: Anticholenergics to decrease secretions and promote relaxation of the gallbladder, analgesics (Dilaudid, morphine), antibiotics, atropine and dicyclomine (Bentyl) will relieve spasms and decrease pain; ketorolac (Toradol) may be used to decrease spasms and pain in older adults. Laparoscopic cholecystectomy.

CHOLELITHIASIS

. . . .

CIRRHOSIS

. . . .

Definition: Presence of stones in the gallbladder; most common form of biliary disease.

Causes: Risk factors and etiology include supersaturation of bile with cholesterol; conditions upsetting cholesterol and bile balance include infection and disturbances of cholesterol metabolism; increased incidence in females, especially during pregnancy, increased occurrence after age 40; obesity.

Assessment Findings: Depends on the mobility of the stone and whether obstruction occurs; epigastric distress; feeling of fullness; abdominal distension; vague pain in the right upper quadrant after consumption of meals high in fat.

Treatment/Nursing Interventions: Cholecystectomy (surgical removal of stones)

. . . .

Definition: A chronic, progressive disease of the liver characterized by diffuse degeneration and destruction of hepatocytes, which causes scar tissue to form. Complications include portal hypertension, ascites, bleeding esophageal varices, coagulation defects, hepatorenal syndrome.

Causes: Chronic alcohol abuse, hepatitis B, hepatitis C, cystic fibrosis, destruction of the bile ducts, fat that accumulates in the liver, hardening and scarring of the bile, galactosemia, hemochromatosis, autoimmune hepatitis, schistosomiasis, biliary atresia, glycogen storage disease.

Assessment Findings: Neurological, GI, renal, endocrine, immune system, cardiovascular, pulmonary, hematologic, dermatologic, and fluid and electrolyte alternations.

Treatment/Nursing Interventions: Elevate the head of the bed, provide supplemental vitamins, restrict sodium and fluid intake as ordered, initiate enteral feedings or parenteral nutrition as ordered; weigh client and measure abdominal girth daily; monitor for asterixis, fector hepaticus, and level of consciousness. Evaluate coagulation laboratory results. Administer diuretics, blood products, antacids, lactulose, antibiotics, as ordered. Maintain gastric intubation to assess bleeding or esophagogastric balloon tamponade to control bleeding. If indicated, prepare client for paracentesis and surgical shunting procedure.

. . . .

PART II

CIRRHOSIS, TYPES OF

. . . .

CROHN'S DISEASE

. . . .

CULLEN'S SIGN

Laennec's Cirrhosis	Alcohol-induced, nutritional, or portal. Cellular necrosis causes eventual widespread scar tissue, with fibrotic infiltration of the liver.
Postnecrotic Cirrhosis	Occurs after massive liver necrosis. Results as a complication of hepatitis or exposure to hepatotoxins. Scar tissue causes destruction of the liver lobules and entire lobes.
Biliary Cirrhosis	Develops from chronic biliary obstruction, bile stasis, and inflammation, resulting in severe obstructive jaundice.
Cardiac Cirrhosis	Associated with severe, right-sided congestive heart failure and results in an enlarged, edematous, congested liver. The liver becomes anoxic, resulting in liver cell necrosis and fibrosis.

Definition: An inflammatory disease that can occur anywhere in the gastrointestinal tract but commonly affects the terminal ileum and leads to thickening and scarring, a narrowed lumen, fistulas, ulcerations, and abscesses.
Causes: High incidence of familiar occurrence.
Assessment Findings: Fever, cramplike and colicky pain after meals, electrolyte imbalances, diarrhea (which may contain mucus and puss), dehydration, anemia, weight loss, anorexia, nausea and vomiting, abdominal dissection, malnutrition, impaired absorption of vitamin B_{12}.
Treatment/Nursing Interventions: Increased calories, protein, and fluid; encourage several small meals each day. Anti-inflammatory: aminosalicylates and corticosteroids. Antimicrobials to prevent and treat infections. Immunosuppressants to decrease or suppress the immune response. Antidiarrheals. Surgical intervention may be necessary if client fails to respond to medical management and if fistulas, perforation, bleeding, or internal obstruction occurs. Total removal of colon, rectum, and anus with the formation of permanent ileostomy and continent ileostomy (Kock's pouch). Minimally invasive surgery (MIS) involves a laparoscopy to remove small areas of diseased tissue in the ileum and ileocecal areas.

Definition: Bluish discoloration of the abdomen and periumbilical area seen in acute hemorrhagic pancreatitis.

NCLEX-RN Flash Review

DIVERTICULITIS

PART II

· ·

ESOPHAGEAL VARICES

· ·

FECTOR HEPATICUS

Definition: Condition in which small pouches or sacs composed of mucous membrane protrude through the muscular wall of the intestine.
Causes: Results from retention of stool and bacteria in the diverticulum. Risk factors include a low-fiber diet; high intake of processed foods, constipation, and indigestible fibers (seeds, corn, etc.) may precipitate the condition, but do not contribute to the development of diverticula.
Assessment Findings: Frequently asymptomatic, but symptoms vary based on the degree inflammation present. Fever, left lower quadrant pain; may be accompanied by nausea and vomiting; abdominal distension and increased pain on palpation.
Treatment/Nursing Interventions: Oral antibiotics, antispasmodic medications, liquid or low-residue diet until better. In its severe form, requires the administration of a broad spectrum antibiotic, bowel rest (NPO, hydration with IV fluid, NG tube placement), pain management with opiates; surgical intervention is required for obstruction, abscess, hemorrhage, or perforation.

· ·

Definition: Tortuous, dilated veins in the submucosa of the lower esophagus, possibly extending into the fundus of the stomach or upward into the esophagus. Bleeding varices are a medical emergency.
Causes: Portal hypertension; often associated with cirrhosis of the liver.
Assessment Findings: Hematemesis, melena, tarry stools, ascites, jaundice, hepatomegaly and splenomegaly, dilated abdominal veins, signs of shock.
Treatment/Nursing Interventions: Monitor vital signs, elevate the head of bed, monitor lung sound, administer oxygen, maintain NPO status, administer IV fluids and electrolytes as ordered, monitor hemoglobin and hematocrit values and coagulation factors, assist in inserting an NG tube or a balloon tamponade if indicated, endoscopic injection, endoscopic variceal ligation, and shunting procedures.

· ·

Definition: An unpleasant odor of the breath in individuals with severe liver disease caused by volatile aromatic substances that accumulate in the blood and urine.

GASTROESOPHAGEAL REFLUX DISEASE (GERD)

....

HEPATITIS

....

HEPATITIS A (HAV)

Definition: Caused by the backward flow and/or reflux of gastric contents into the esophagus. Amount of damage experienced depends on the amount and composition of gastric contents, as well as the ability of the esophagus to remove the acid fluid.

Causes: Risk factors include obesity, smoking, excess alcohol intake, consumption of high-fat meals, consumption of caffeine and carbonated beverages, stress.

Assessment Findings: Heartburn, dyspepsia, regurgitation not associated with bleeding or nausea, increased discomfort/pain following meals that may be alleviated with antacids, and pain that radiates to the back and neck; activities that increase intra-abdominal pressure increase esophageal discomfort.

Treatment/Nursing Interventions: Diet therapy involves avoiding the intake of fatty foods; eating small, frequent meals; chewing gum after and between meals; avoiding wine and other alcoholic beverages, caffeinated drinks, and chocolate. Medication may include histamine-2 receptors antagonists, proton pump inhibitors, and GI stimulants or promotility medications. Surgical interventions involve fundoplication or antireflux surgery. Endoscopic intervention at lower esophagus and gastroesophageal sphincter (fundoplication, radiofrequency, sclerosing agents).

. . . .

Definition: An inflammation of the liver that can be caused by a group of viruses. There are five major types of viral hepatitis: A, B, C, D, E. Types A, B, and C are the most common.

. . . .

Description: Formally known as infectious hepatitis; seen in fall and early winter.

Individuals at Risk: Young children; individuals in institutional settings; healthcare personnel.

Transmission: Fecal-oral route; person-to-person contact; parenteral; contaminated fruits, vegetables, or uncooked shellfish; contaminated water or milk; poorly washed utensils.

Incubation and Infectious Period: Incubation period is 2 to 6 weeks; infectious period is 2 to 3 weeks before and 1 week after development of jaundice.

Testing: Presence of HAV antibodies in blood; increased levels of immunoglobulin M (IgM) in the blood.

Complications: Fulminant (severe acute and often fatal) hepatitis.

Prevention: Strict hand washing; stool precautions; treatment of municipal water supplies; serological screening of food handlers; hepatitis A vaccine (Havrix VAQTA).

HEPATITIS B (HBV)

· ·

HEPATITIS C (HCV)

· ·

HIATAL HERNIA

PART
II

Description: Nonseasonal; all age groups are affected.
Individuals at Risk: IV drug users; clients undergoing long-term hemodialysis; healthcare personnel.
Transmission: Blood or bloody fluid contact; infected blood products; infected saliva or semen; contaminated needles; sexual contact; parenteral; perinatal; blood, bloody fluid, or body fluids contact at birth.
Incubation Period: 6 to 24 weeks.
Testing: Presence of hepatitis B antigen-antibody systems in the blood; presence of hepatitis B surface antigen (HBsAG) in the blood.
Complications: Fulminant hepatitis; chronic liver disease; cirrhosis; primary hepatocellular carcinoma.
Prevention: Strict hand washing; screening blood donors; testing of all pregnant women; needle precautions; avoiding intimate sexual contact with hepatitis B carriers; hepatitis B vaccine (Engerix-B for adults; Recombivax for children).

. . . .

Description: Occurs year-round; occurs in any age group; is the major cause of posttransfusion hepatitis.
Individuals at Risk: IV drug users; clients receiving frequent blood transfusions.
Transmission: Same as HBV, primarily through blood.
Incubation Period: 5 to 10 weeks.
Testing: Presence of anti-HVC in the blood.
Complications: Chronic liver disease; cirrhosis; primary hepatocellular carcinoma.
Prevention: Strict hand washing; screening of blood donors; needle precautions.

. . . .

Definition: Protrusion of a portion of the stomach through the diaphragm and into the thorax. Also known as esophageal or diaphragmatic hernia.
Causes: Congenital weakness, trauma, relaxation of muscles, increased intra-abdominal pressure.
Assessment Findings: Heartburn, dyspepsia, feeling of fullness, regurgitating or vomiting.
Treatment/Nursing Interventions: Medical and surgical management are similar to those for GERD; avoid anticholinergics (which delay stomach emptying); eat small, frequent meals and limit the amount of liquids taken with meals; advise client not to recline for 1 hour after eating.
Special Considerations: Complications include ulceration, hemorrhage, regurgitation and aspiration of stomach content, strangulation, and incarceration of the stomach in the chest with possible necrosis, peritonitis, and mediastinitis.

JAUNDICE

· ·

MURPHY'S SIGN

· ·

PANCREATITIS

PART
II

Definition: A yellow color of the skin, mucus membranes, or eyes. The yellow coloring comes from bilirubin, a by-product of old red blood cells. Occurs when too many red blood cells are dying or breaking down and going to the liver, the liver is overloaded or damaged, or the bilirubin from the liver is unable to move through the digestive tract properly. Commonly a sign of liver, gallbladder, or pancreas problems. Infections, use of certain medications, cancer, blood disorders, gallstones, birth defects, and a number of other medical conditions can lead to this condition.

• •

Definition: Indicates inflammation of the gallbladder. The client is asked to inhale while the examiner's fingers are positioned under the liver border at the bottom of the rib cage. The inspiration causes the gallbladder to descend onto the fingers, producing pain. Deep inspiration is limited.

• •

Definition: An inflammatory condition of the pancreas. The acute form is characterized by an inflammatory process; problems range from mild edema to severe hypotension and severe hemorrhagic necrosis. In contrast, the chronic form is characterized by progressive destruction and fibrosis of the pancreas.

Causes: Risk factors include trauma; certain medications (thiazide diuretics, NSAIDs, estrogen, steroids, salicylates); hyperlipidemia; biliary tract disease, causing reflux of bile secretions; alcohol intake, precipitating an increase in the secretion of pancreatic enzymes.

Assessment Findings: *General:* Severe constant midepigastric pain that radiates to the back or flank area and is exacerbated by eating. *Acute:* Persistent vomiting, low-grade fever, hypotension and tachycardia, jaundice, abdominal distention, Cullen's sign, Grey Turner's sign. *Chronic:* Decrease in weight, mild jaundice, steatorrhea, abdominal distention and tenderness, hyperglycemia.

Treatment/Nursing Interventions: Administration of antibiotics and analgesics. Interventions are directed at decreasing pancreatic stimulus: NPO status, administration of IV fluids, nasogastric suction, bed rest; low-fat, high-carbohydrate diet if not NPO. Surgical intervention may be required to eliminate precipitating cause (biliary obstruction).

NCLEX-RN Flash Review

PEPTIC ULCER DISEASE (PUD)

. . . .

PERISTALSIS

. . . .

PORTAL HYPERTENSION

Definition: An erosion of the GI mucosa by hydrochloric acid and pepsin. Any location in the GI tract that comes in contact with gastric secretions is susceptible. There are three types: duodenal (most common), gastric, and physiologic stress ulcers.

Causes: Predisposing factors include stress, smoking, the use of alcohol, NSAIDs, corticosteroids, history of gastritis, infection with *H. pylori*, family history of gastric ulcers.

Assessment Findings: Burning pain lasting minutes to hours; the pain associated with ulcers can overlap and can be confusing. *Gastric type:* Pain is high in the epigastric area; occurs 1 to 2 hours after eating. *Duodenal type:* Pain is in the midepigastric area just below the xiphoid process, or in the back; occurs 2 to 4 hours after eating and is relieved by antacids or eating.

Treatment/Nursing Interventions: Dependent on client presentation and presence of complications (hemorrhage, perforation, gastric outlet obstruction). General medications: Metronidazole (Flagyl), omeprazole (Omeprazile, Prilosec), clarithromycin, amoxicillin, and tetracycline (all used to eliminate *H. pylori* bacteria). Additional medications: antacids, histamine-2 receptor (H2R) antagonists, prostaglandin analogs, and proton pump inhibitors (PPIs).

Special Considerations: Often results in an emergency situation—may initially be treated conservatively; however, surgery may be required. Hot, spicy, or rough foods are not factors associated with PUD.

• •

Definition: Wavelike rhythmic contractions that propel material through the gastrointestinal tract.

• •

Definition: An increase in the pressure within the portal vein (the vein that carries blood from the digestive organs to the liver).

Causes: The increase in pressure is caused by a blockage in the blood flow through the liver. Increased pressure in the portal vein causes large veins (varices) to develop across the esophagus and stomach to bypass the blockage. The varices become fragile and can bleed easily. Results from cirrhosis or scarring of the liver.

Assessment Findings: Gastrointestinal bleeding; black, tarry stools or bloody stools; or vomiting of blood due to the spontaneous rupture and hemorrhage from varices; ascites, encephalopathy, and reduced levels of platelets or decreased white blood cell count.

TURNER'S SIGN

. . . .

ULCERATIVE COLITIS

. . . .

Definition: A gray-blue discoloration of the flank seen in acute hemorrhagic pancreatitis.

. . . .

Definition: An inflammatory bowel disease (IBD) that causes chronic inflammation of the digestive tract; characterized by abdominal pain and diarrhea. Usually affects only the innermost lining of the large intestine (colon) and rectum.

Causes: Can occur at any age, but often affects people in their 30s. Some people may not develop the disease until their 50s or 60s; Caucasians have the highest risk of the disease; family history, altered immune response are also implicated.

Assessment Findings: Rectal bleeding, diarrhea; increased stools (10–20) per day during an acute exacerbation; fever, malaise, anorexia; tenesmus.

Treatment/Nursing Interventions: Increased calories, protein, and fluid; encourage several small meals each day. Administration of aminosalicylates and corticosteroids to decrease inflammation as ordered. Surgical intervention may be necessary if client fails to respond to medical management and if fistulas, perforation, bleeding, or internal obstruction occur. Total removal of colon, rectum, and anus with the formation of permanent ileostomy or continent ileostomy (Kock's pouch); laparoscopy can be performed to remove small areas of diseased tissue in the ileum and ileocecal areas.

. . . .

ACUTE TRANSFUSION REACTIONS

PART II

· ·

ANEMIA

· ·

Reaction	Clinical Manifestation
Acute Hemolytic	Chills, fever, lower back pain, tachycardia, dyspnea, tachypnea, hypotension, vascular collapse, acute jaundice, bleeding, shock, cardiac arrest, death
Febrile/Nonhemolytic (most common)	Sudden chill and fever, headache, flushing, anxiety, vomiting, muscle pain
Mild Allergic	Flushing, itching, hives
Anaphylactic and Severe Allergic	Anxiety, urticaria, dyspnea, wheezing, progressing to cyanosis, bronchospasms, hypotension, shock, possible cardiac arrest
Circulatory Overload	Cough, dyspnea, pulmonary congestion, headache, hypertension, tachycardia, distended neck veins
Sepsis	Rapid onset of chills, high fever, vomiting, diarrhea, hypotension, shock

• •

Definition: A condition that occurs in which either quality or quantity of blood decreases. Deficiency may be a decrease in erythrocytes or a lower than normal level of hemoglobin.

Causes: Acute or chronic blood loss, destruction of red blood cells, abnormal bone marrow function, drugs, chemicals, chemotherapy, decreased erythpoietin due to renal damage, subtherapeutic maturation of red blood cells.

Assessment Findings: Weakness and fatigue, lethargy, dyspnea, tachycardia, tachypnea, pallor, cold extremities, vertigo, irritability, depression, poor healing, vertigo.

Treatment/Nursing Interventions: Provide a diet high in protein, iron, and vitamins, maintain adequate fluid intake, provide bed rest as necessary, protect from injury, avoid extremes of cold or heat, provide mouth care with diluted mouthwash and soft toothbrush, provide emotional support for long-term therapy.

• •

ANEMIA, APLASTIC

. . . .

ANEMIA, IRON-DEFICIENCY

. . . .

Definition: A deficiency of marrow stem cells as a result of bone marrow suppression. Pancytopenia (deficiency of all types of blood cells, including white blood cells, red blood cells, and platelets) often accompanies red blood cell (RBC) deficiency.

Causes: Exposure to radiation and chemotherapy, chemicals (DDT, benzene), medications (Dilantin, chloromycetin, sulfonamides, alkylating agents, anticonvulsants [Mesantoin]), viral infection, pregnancy, diseases that suppress bone marrow activity (leukemia and metastatic cancer).

Assessment Findings: Fatigue, shortness of breath with exertion, rapid or irregular heart rate, pale skin, frequent or prolonged infections, un-explained or easy bruising, nosebleeds and bleeding gums, prolonged bleeding from cuts, skin rash, dizziness, headache.

Treatment/Nursing Interventions: Transfusion of RCBs and/or platelets, stem cell transplant, administration of androgens and/or corticosteroids, and antibiotics as ordered. Protect from infection, place client in private room, and prevent fatigue.

. . . .

Definition: The most common type of anemia, slowly progressive, related to an iron deficiency. Frequently occurs in infants, adolescents, pregnant females, alcoholics, and the elderly.

Causes: Chronic blood loss, inadequate nutritional intake, defective absorption, improper utilization of iron, prolonged drug therapy, improper cooking of foods.

Assessment Findings: Cheilosis, extertional dyspnea, glossitis, papillae atrophy of tongue; check for pica syndrome; concave, brittle nails; fatigue and lack of energy.

Treatment/Nursing Interventions: Provide foods high in iron, administer iron preparations as prescribed: *Oral:* Ferrous sulfate; provide liquid iron with a straw (stains teeth); iron oral supplements should be taken on an empty stomach; give iron with orange juice or vitamin C, as this aids in absorption; watch for and educate client about the side effects of iron: constipation, nausea and diarrhea, abdominal cramps, epigastric distress; alert clients that stool will be black. *Parenteral:* Administer Imferon (IV, IM), Sorbitex (IM), using the z-track method of administration. Monitor fluid and electrolyte balance; provide frequent rest periods for intense fatigue.

. . . .

ANEMIA, MEGALOBLASTIC

. . . .

BLOOD PRODUCTS I

. . . .

Definition: Type of anemia involving morphologic changes that are caused by defective DNA synthesis and abnormal RBC maturation.

Causes: Primary cause is deficiency of vitamin B_{12} or folic acid. Absence of intrinsic factor, surgical resection of the stomach, alcohol abuse and anorexia infections, atrophy of the gastric mucosa, malabsorption syndrome/disease, bacterial or parasitic infections. *Medications:* Methotrexate, oral contraceptives, and anticonvulsants.

Assessment Findings: Yellow cast to the skin, pallor, tingling of the extremities (which does not occur with folic acid deficiency), peripheral neuropathy, weakness, fatigue, anorexia, personality and behavioral changes, beefy/red tongue (glossitis), alterations in gait (loss of balance).

Treatment/Nursing Interventions: Serum blood work for RBC count and megaloblastic maturation; administer B_{12} deep IM (usually once a month); change amount of dietary intake and oral folic acid if anemia is caused by folic acid deficiency due to chronic alcoholism; provide safety measures if neurological alterations are observed. Prepare client for possible bone marrow aspiration, upper GI series, gastric analysis, Schilling test, and/or gastric analysis.

Product	Description	Indications for Usage
Packed RBCs	Prepared from whole blood by sedimentation or centrifugation (one unit contains 250–300 mL).	Anemia, acute blood loss.
Frozen RBCs	Prepared from RBCs using glycerol for protection and freezing; they can be stored for ten years at 188.6°F.	Autotransfusion; stockpiling or rare donors for clients with alloantibodies. Not often used because filters remove most white blood cells (WBCs).
Platelets	Prepared from fresh whole blood within 4 hours after collection.	Bleeding caused by thrombocytopenia, may be contraindicated in immune thrombocytopenia purpura, thrombotic thrombocytopenic purpura, and heparin-induced thrombocytopenia except in life-threatening situations.

BLOOD PRODUCTS II

. . . .

**INTRAMUSCULAR MEDICATION
ADMINISTRATION: Z-TRACK METHOD**

. . . .

Product	Description	Indications for Usage
Fresh-Frozen Plasma	Liquid portion of blood is separated from cells and frozen. Plasma is rich in clotting factors but contains no platelets. It can be stored for 1 year and must be used 2 hours after thawing.	Bleeding caused by deficiency in clotting factors.
Albumin	Prepared from plasma. It can be stored for 5 years.	Hypovolemic shock, hypoalbuminemia.
Cryopre-cipitate and Commercial Concentra-tions	Prepared from fresh plasma with 10–20 mL/bag. It can be stored for 1 year and once thawed must be used immediately.	Replacement of clotting factors, especially factor VIII, von Willebrand disease, and fibrinogen.

1. Draw up the medication in the syringe using aseptic technique.

2. Add 0.25 mL of air to the syringe.

3. Discard the needle used to draw up the medication.

4. Place a new 22-gauge (2–3 inches) long needle on the syringe.

5. Select the dorsal gluteal site for the injection.

6. Once the site is selected, pull the skin and subcutaneous tissue sideways away from the muscle.

7. Cleanse the site while holding the skin and subcutaneous tissue off to the side.

8. Insert the needle deeply into the muscle tissue.

9. Aspirate to determine needle placement.

10. If blood is aspirated, withdraw the needle and begin the procedure again from the beginning.

11. If no blood is aspirated, inject the medication slowly, followed by the injection of the air bubble.

12. Quickly withdraw the needle.

13. Release the skin and subcutaneous tissue—do not massage injection site.

NCLEX-RN Flash Review

LEUKEMIA

· ·

POLYCYTHEMIA

· ·

Definition: Malignant disorder of blood-forming tissue (including bone marrow and lymphatic system) characterized by neoplastic proliferation of hematopoietic cells or their precursors. Classification is based on its speed of progression and the type of cells involved. In acute type, abnormal blood cells are immature blood cells (blasts). Chronic type involves more mature blood cells, which produce no symptoms and can go undiagnosed for years.
Causes: Thought to be a combination of genetic and environmental factors. Predisposing factors include excess radiation exposure, viral factors, bone marrow alterations, immune alterations, noxious chemicals, and drugs.
Assessment Findings: Fever or chills, persistent fatigue, weakness, frequent infections, unexplained weight loss, swollen lymph nodes, enlarged liver or spleen, easy bleeding or bruising, petechiae, excessive sweating (especially at night), bone pain or tenderness.
Treatment/Nursing Interventions: Chemotherapy, preventing complications of medications, maintaining fluid and electrolyte balance, providing high-calorie and high-protein diet, providing emotional support and client education, and preventing infection, hemorrhage, and ulceration.
Special Considerations: Major types: acute lymphocytic leukemia (ALL), mostly in young children; acute myelogenous leukemia (AML), occurs in children and adults; chronic lymphocytic leukemia (CLL), most common adult leukemia, very rare in children; and chronic myelogenous leukemia (CML), mainly affects adults.

· ·

Definition: A condition that results in an increased level of circulating red blood cells in the bloodstream. This disorder also causes an increase in hematocrit (HCT), hemoglobin (HGB), or red blood cell counts. Normally discussed in terms of increased hematocrit or hemoglobin.
HCT: Disorder considered when the hematocrit is greater than 48% in women and 52% in men.
HGB: Disorder considered when the hemoglobin level is greater than 16.5 g/dL in women and greater than 18.5 g/dL in men.
Can be divided into two categories: primary and secondary. In primary form, the increase in red blood cells is due to inherent problems in the process of red blood cell production. In secondary form, the increase generally occurs as a response to other factors or underlying conditions that promote red blood cell production.

· ·

THROMBOCYTOPENIA

Definition: Any disorder in which there is an abnormally low number of platelets. Often divided into three major causes of low platelets: low production of platelets in the bone marrow, increased breakdown of platelets in the bloodstream, and increased breakdown of platelets in the spleen or liver.

Disorders that involve low production in the bone marrow include aplastic anemia, cancer in the bone marrow, cirrhosis, folate deficiency, and vitamin B$_{12}$ deficiency. The use of certain medications and chemotherapy treatments may also lead to a low production of platelets in the bone marrow.

BURNS, CAUSES OF

. . . .

BURNS, CHEMICAL: EMERGENCY MANAGEMENT

. . . .

BURNS, ELECTRICAL: EMERGENCY MANAGEMENT

Type	Source
Thermal	Excessive heat from fire, flames, hot liquids, hot objects, steam
Electrical	Lightning, electrical current
Chemical	Acids, bases, caustics
Radiation	Ultraviolet light, nuclear radiation
Light	Sunlight, ultraviolet light
Inhalation	Inhalation of air or noxious chemicals (two types: smoke inhalation, inhalation of carbon dioxide)

• •

Causes: Alkalis, acids, organic compounds.
Assessment Findings: Burning, localized pain, redness, swelling of injured tissue, paralysis, degeneration of exposed tissue, discoloration of injured skin, edema of surrounding tissues, respiratory distress (if chemical inhaled).
Nursing Interventions: *Initial:* Secure patent airway; cervical spine stabilization; anticipate intubation with significant inhalation injury, circumferential full-thickness burns to the neck/chest, and or large total body surface area (TBSA) burn; assess airway, breathing, and circulation before decontamination procedures; brush dry chemical from skin before irrigation; flush chemical; remove nonadherent clothing, shoes, watches, jewelry, glasses, or contact lenses when face is exposed; initiate fluid replacement; insert urinary catheter; elevate burned limbs; administer IV pain medications as ordered; cover burned areas with dry dressings or clean sheet. *Ongoing care:* Monitor airway; monitor urinary output.

• •

Causes: Electric and utility wires; lightning; defibrillator.
Assessment Findings: Lethargy, white or charred skin, burn odor, impaired touch or sensation, minimal pain or sensation, dysrhythmias, location of contact points, decreased peripheral circulation if extremities injured, thermal burns if clothes ignite, fractures or dislocations from current or force, head or neck injury if associated with fall, depth and extent of wound difficult to visualize; always assume injury is greater than what is observed.
Nursing Interventions: *Initial:* Secure patient airway; cervical spine stabilization; assess and monitor vital signs, level of consciousness, oxygen saturation, and cardiac rhythm; assess airway, breathing, and circulation; remove nonadherent clothing, shoes, watches, jewelry, glasses, or contact lenses when face is exposed; initiate fluid replacement; insert urinary catheter; elevate burned limbs above heart to decrease edema; administer IV pain medications; treat associated injuries; cover burned areas with dry dressing or clean sheet. *Ongoing care:* Monitor airway, urinary output/urine for the development of myoglobinuria, vital signs, level of consciousness, oxygen saturation, and cardiac rhythm; anticipate the administration of mannitol and $NaHCO_3$ and hemoglobinuria.

BURNS, THERMAL: EMERGENCY MANAGEMENT

....

BURN DEPTH I

....

Causes: Hot liquids or solids; flash flame; open flame; steam; hot surface; ultraviolet rays.

Assessment Findings: *Partial thickness (superficial):* redness, pain, moderate to severe tenderness, blanching with pressure. *Partial thickness (deep):* Moist blebs, blisters; mottled white, pink, cherry red; hypersensitive to touch or air; moderate to severe pain; blanching with pressure. *Full thickness:* Dry, leathery eschar; white waxy, dark brown, or charred appearance; burn odor (strong); impaired sensation when touched. Absence of pain with severe pain in surrounding tissues; lack of blanching with pressure.

Nursing Interventions: *Initial:* Secure patent airway; cervical spine stabilization; assess for inhalation injury; assess and monitor vital signs, level of consciousness, oxygen saturation, and cardiac rhythm; assess airway, breathing, and circulation; remove nonadherent clothing, shoes, watches, jewelry, glasses, or contact lenses when face is exposed; initiate fluid replacement; insert urinary catheter; elevate burned limb; administer IV pain medications; treat associated injuries; cover burned areas with dry dressing or clean sheet. *Ongoing care:* Monitor airway, urinary output, vital signs, level of consciousness, oxygen saturation, and cardiac rhythm.

Depth	Description
Superficial Thickness Burn	Limited to the epidermis, skin blanches with pressure, painful, skin appears red, requires local wound care, no scarring occurs, heals in 3–6 days (example: sunburn).
Superficial Partial-Thickness Burn	Injury into the dermis, large blisters, edema, mottled pink to red base and broken epidermis, with a wet, shiny, and weeping surface, painful and sensitive to cold air, heals in 10–21 days with no scarring, grafts may be used if the healing process is prolonged.
Deep Partial-Thickness Burn	Expands deeper into the skin dermis, blister formation usually does not occur because the dead tissue layer is thick and sticks to underlying viable dermis. Wound surface is red and dry with white areas in deeper parts, may or may not blanch, moderate edema, heals in 3–6 weeks, scar formation occurs.

BURN DEPTH II

PART
II

. . . .

FLUID RESUSCITATION FORMULAS: FIRST 24 HOURS FOLLOWING A BURN INJURY

. . . .

Depth	Description
Full-Thickness Burn	Injury and destruction of the epidermis and the dermis; the wound will not heal by reepithelialization, and grafting may be necessary. Skin appears as dry, hard, leathery eschar, which is waxy white, deep red, yellow, brown, or black in color. Sensation is reduced or absent due to nerve ending destruction. Healing may take weeks to months and depends on establishing adequate blood supply; burn requires eschar removal and grafting; if not prevented, scarring and wound contractures may develop.
Deep Full-Thickness Burn	Injury extends beyond the skin into underlying fascia and tissues, and muscle, bone, and tendons are damaged. Injured areas appear black and sensation is completely absent. Eschar is hard and inelastic. Healing takes months, and grafts are required.

· ·

Formula	Solution	Rate of Administration
Modified Brooke 0.5 mL to 15 mL/kg/% TBSA Burn	• Protenate or 5% albumin in isotonic saline • Lactated Ringer's (LR) without dextrose	• Half given in the first 8 hours • Half given in the next 16 hours
Parkland (Baxter) 4 mL/kg/% TBSA Burn	• Crystalloid only—LR	• Half given in the first 8 hours, half given in the next 16 hours
Modified Parkland 4 mL/kg/% TBSA Burn + 15mL/m² of TBSA	• Crystalloid only—LR	• Half given in the first 8 hours, half given in the next 16 hours

TBSA = Total body surface area.

· ·

HERPES ZOSTER (SHINGLES)

. . . .

INHALATION INJURY: EMERGENCY MANAGEMENT

. . . .

Definition: A painful, blistering skin rash due to the varicella-zoster virus, which causes chickenpox. The virus remains inactive (becomes dormant) in certain nerves in the body, and becomes active again in the nerves years later. May develop in any age group, but more likely to develop in those who are older than 60, who had chickenpox before age 1, and who have immune systems weakened by medications or disease. If adults or children have direct contact with the shingles rash on someone and have not had chickenpox as a child or a chickenpox vaccine, they can develop chickenpox, rather than shingles. The first symptom is usually one-sided pain, tingling, or burning. The pain and burning may be severe and are usually present before any rash appears.

· ·

Causes: Exposure to intense heat or flames; inhalation of carbon monoxide, noxious chemicals, or smoke; client burned in an enclosed space or clothing catching fire.

Assessment Findings: Shallow, rapid respirations; oxygen saturation, hoarseness, coughing; singed facial or nasal hair, black/darkened oral/nasal membranes; smoky breath, carbonaceous sputum; cough with black, gray, or bloody sputum; difficulty swallowing; altered mental status.

Nursing Interventions: *Initial:* Secure patent airway; cervical spine stabilization; assess for inhalation injury; assess and monitor vital signs, level of consciousness, oxygen saturation, and cardiac rhythm; assess airway, breathing, and circulation; remove nonadherent clothing, shoes, watches, jewelry, glasses, or contact lenses when face is exposed; initiate fluid replacement; insert urinary catheter; obtain ABG, carboxyhemoglobin levels, and chest x-ray; administer IV pain medications; treat associated injuries; cover burned areas with dry dressing or clean sheet; anticipate need for fiberoptic bronchoscopy or intubation. *Ongoing care:* Monitor airway, urinary output, vital signs, level of consciousness, oxygen saturation, and cardiac rhythm.

· ·

PRESSURE ULCERS, STAGES OF

· ·

RULE OF NINES

· ·

Stage	Description
Stage I	• Intact skin • Nonblanching erythema
Stage II	• Epidermis interrupted • Dermis may be interrupted • Abrasion or blister
Stage III	• Full thickness • Damage and/or necrosis down to the fascia
Stage IV	• Full thickness • Penetrates the fascia • Involves muscle, tendon, and/or bone

Method to Estimate Extent of Burn Injury

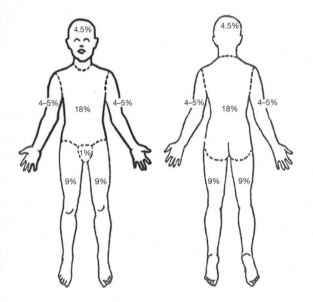

NCLEX-RN Flash Review

AMPUTATION

. . . .

CRUTCH WALKING

. . . .

CRUTCH WALKING: GOING UP STAIRS

Definition: Surgical removal of a diseased part or organ.
Causes: Peripheral vascular disease (PVD) (80% to 75% of which are diabetic clients); trauma; infection; congenital deformities; malignant tumors.
Assessment Findings: Prior to amputation, assessment findings of PVD include decreased pain/feeling in the affected extremity, cool extremity, leathery skin on affected extremity, absent peripheral pulses, hair loss on affected extremity, necrotic tissue or wounds (area blue or blue-gray turning black, drainage possible, with or without odor).
Treatment/Nursing Interventions: Provide wound care; monitor surgical dressing for drainage; mark dressing for bleeding; measure suction drainage; change dressing as ordered; monitor for signs of infection; elevate residual limb (stump) for 24 hours postoperatively; position client to decrease edema and spasms of the stump; be aware of phantom pain that is real pain; provide passive range of motion (ROM); collaborate with rehabilitation team for mobility needs; handle affected stump gently; encourage independence in self-care.

· ·

Non-Weight-Bearing—Placing no weight on the injured leg.

1. Instruct the client to place the crutches forward about one step's length while pushing down on the hand grips.

2. Instruct the client to squeeze the top of the crutches between the body and the upper arm while holding the injured leg up from the floor.

3. Instruct the client to swing the good leg forward, while being careful not to go too far.

4. Instruct the client to now step on the good leg and bring crutches forward to one step's length.

· ·

1. Instruct the client to face the stairs squarely.

2. Instruct the client to place both crutches close to the first step.

3. Instruct the client to put the uninjured leg on the first step.

4. Instruct the client to push from the strong leg, and lift both crutches and the injured leg up to the step.

5. Instruct the client to repeat the sequence for each step.

PART II

FRACTURE

. . . .

FRACTURES, COMPLICATIONS OF, I

. . . .

FRACTURES, COMPLICATIONS OF, II

Definition: A break in the continuity of the bone caused by trauma, twisting as a result of muscle spasm or indirect loss of leverage, or bone decalcification and disease that result in osteopenia.

Assessment Findings: pain and tenderness over the involved area; loss or decrease in muscular strength or function; muscle spasm and neurovascular impairment; obvious deformity of affected area; crepitation, erythema, edema, bruising.

Treatment/Nursing Interventions: Reduction, fixation, traction, and casting; emergency/initial care involves immobilization of the affected extremity with casting or splinting; assessment of neurovascular status of the extremity.

Complication	Description
Pulmonary Embolism	Caused by the movement of foreign particles (blood clot, fat, or air) into the pulmonary circulation. *Assessment findings:* Restlessness, apprehensiveness, dyspnea, chest pain, cough, hemoptysis, hypoxemia, crackles.
Avascular Necrosis	Occurs when the fracture interrupts blood supply to a section of the bone, resulting in bone death. *Assessment findings:* Decreased sensation and pain.
Fat Embolism	Originates in the bone marrow and occurs after a fracture when a fat globule is released into the bloodstream. Prevalence is higher in clients with a long bone fracture. Can occur 48 to 72 hours following an injury. *Assessment findings:* Restlessness, hypoxemia, mental status changes, tachycardia, hypotension, dyspnea, tachypnea, petechial rash over the upper chest and neck, which may fade quickly.

Complication	Description
Infection and Osteomyelitis	These complications can be caused by the introduction of organisms into the bones, leading to localized bone infection. *Assessment findings:* Tachycardia; fever (above 101°F); erythema and pain in the area surrounding the infection; leukocytosis and elevated erythrocyte sedimentation rate (ESR).
Compartment Syndrome	Tough fascia surrounds muscle groups, forming compartments from which arteries, veins, and nerves enter and exit at opposite ends. Occurs when pressure in one or more compartments is increased and results in decreased blood flow, tissue ischemia, and neurovascular impairment. *Assessment findings:* Unrelieved or increased pain in the affected limb; pulselessness (late); paresthesia; pain with passive movement; tissue that is distal to the involved area becomes pale, dusky, or edematous.

FRACTURES, HIP, FEMORAL NECK

PART II

. . . .

FRACTURES, HIP, INTERTROCHANTERIC

. . . .

Description: *Intrascapular:* femoral head is broken within the joint capsule.
Assessment Findings: Femoral head and neck receive decreased blood supply and heal slowly; history of slight trauma; pain in the groin and hip; commonly occurs in women ≥60 years of age; lateral rotation and shortening of leg with minimal deformity.
Treatment/Nursing Interventions: Femoral head replacement with prosthesis, threaded pins; total hip replacement or open reduction with internal fixation (ORIF) with femoral replacement. To prevent hip displacement postoperatively, avoid extreme hip flexion.
Possible Complications: Avascular necrosis of femoral head; nonunion; pin complications; dislocation of prosthesis.

. . . .

Description: *Extracapsular:* fracture is outside the joint capsule.
Assessment Findings: Fracture can occur at the greater trochanter or can be an intertrochanteric fracture; history of direct trauma over trochanter; occurs in women usually between the ages of 60 and 85; can occur in younger women with osteoporosis; external rotation and shortening of leg with obvious deformity; loss of hip motion.
Treatment/Nursing Interventions: Open reduction: internal fixation with nail, pin, compression plate with screw. Preoperative treatment includes balanced suspension or skin traction to relieve muscle spasms and reduce pain.
Possible Complications: Shortening of the leg; traumatic arthritis; pin migration; bending or breaking of pin; fracture impaction; loss reduction; delayed union or nonunion of bone.

. . . .

FRACTURES, TYPES OF

. . . .

GOUT

. . . .

Type	Description
Closed or Simple	Skin over area remains intact.
Comminuted	Bone is splintered or crushed, creating numerous fragments.
Complete	Bone is separated completely by a break into two parts.
Compression	Fractured bone is compressed by other bone.
Depressed	Bone fragments are driven inward.
Greenstick	One side of the bone is broken and the other is bent; occurs most commonly in children.
Impacted	Part of the fractured bone is driven into another bone.
Incomplete	Fracture line does not extend through the full transverse width of the bone.
Oblique	Fracture line runs at an angle across the axis of the bone.
Open or Compounded	Bone is exposed to air through a break in the skin.
Pathological	Results from weakening of the bone structure by pathological processes such as neoplasia or osteomalacia; also called spontaneous fracture.
Spiral	Break partially encircles bone.
Transverse	Break is straight across the bone

Definition: Condition in which urate crystals and infiltrating leukocytes damage intracellular phagolysosomes, causing leakage of lysomal enzymes into the synovial fluid, which causes tissue damage and joint inflammation.
Causes: Risk factors include male gender; age ≥50 years; genetic/familial tendency; prolonged hyperuricemia (elevated serum uric acid level).
Assessment Findings: Pain described as "excruciating"; fatigue; anorexia; joints appear with erythema, hot and swollen, difficult to move, skin stretched and shiny over joint; subcutaneous nodules, trophy (deposits of urate) on hands and feet; weight loss; fever; sensory changes, with cold intolerance. Elevated serum uric acid levels; elevated serum WBC; erythrocyte sedimentation rate ≥20mm/hr; proteinuria; azotemia.
Treatment/Nursing Interventions: Administer antigout medication as ordered (Colchicine, phenylbutazone/Butazolidin, Indomethacin/Indocin, allopurinol/Zyloprin); absolute rest of affected joint, then gradual increase in activities; prevent kidney damage; increase fluid intake to 2,000–3,000 mL/day unless contraindicated; monitor urinary output; instruct the client on the importance of a low-purine diet during acute attacks; instruct on dosage and side effects of medications.

OSTEOMYELITIS

· ·

OSTEOPOROSIS

· ·

Definition: An infection of the bone, bone marrow, and surrounding soft tissue. Causative organism is commonly *Staphylococcus aureus*. Initially an inflammatory response occurs with increased vascularization and edema. Even though the healing process occurs, the dead bone tissue frequently forms a sequestrum, which continues to retain bacteria; this tissue may produce recurrent abscesses for years. Classified as acute (sudden onset; may heal in 2 to 3 weeks, or subsequently progress to the chronic form), or chronic (a continuous, persistent problem or exacerbation of previous problem).

Causes: Indirect entry of organism: hematogenous; direct injury (trauma; surgical procedures), which can occur at any age.

Assessment Findings: *Acute:* tenderness, swelling, and warmth; constant pain in the affected area; drainage from infected site; fever; chills; nausea; night sweats; circulatory impairment. *Chronic* (lasts longer than a month; failed to respond to initial course of antibiotic therapy): drainage from sinus tract or wound; recurrent episodes of bone pain; low-grade fever; local signs of infection.

Treatment/Nursing Interventions: IV or oral antibiotic for 6 to 8 weeks; immobilization of affected area; surgical debridement if indicated; hyperbaric oxygen therapy to stimulate circulation and healing.

. . . .

Definition: Decrease in the amount of bone capable of maintaining structural integrity of the skeleton. Loss of bone mass associated with aging increases fragility and risk of fractures.

Causes: Bone remodeling results in increased bone mass until age 35; thereafter, bone mass decreases; lack of vitamin D; calcium deficiency; low estrogen levels after menopause, excessive intake of corticosteroids, malabsorption, lactose intolerance, alcohol abuse, renal failure.

Assessment Findings: Back pain radiating to the trunk, skeletal deformities, pathological fractures. Monitor serum calcium, phosphorus, and alkaline phosphatase levels (usually normal); parathyroid hormones may be elevated.

Treatment/Nursing Interventions: Provide pain control; prevent fractures; administer medications as ordered: estrogen replacement, calcium, calcitonin, fluoride, Fosamax, vitamin D. Instruct the client about the importance of a regular exercise program that includes ROM and weight-bearing exercises and ambulation several times per day. Provide a diet high in protein, calcium, and vitamin D, and express the need to avoid alcohol and coffee.

. . . .

REDUCTION, TYPES OF

. . . .

RHEUMATOID ARTHRITIS

. . . .

Type	Description
Closed	• Manual realignment of bone fragments to previous anatomic position. • Traction and countertraction are manually applied to bone fragments to restore position, length, and alignment. • Completed while client is under local or general anesthesia. • After reduction, traction, casting, external fixation, splints, or orthoses (braces), immobilize injured part to maintain alignment until healing occurs.
Open	• Correction of bone alignment through surgical incision. • Normally includes internal fixation of the fracture with wires, screws, pins, plates, intramedullary rods, or nails. • If open reduction with internal fixation (ORIF) is utilized for intra-articular fractures (involving joint surfaces), early initiation of ROM is necessary.
Traction	• Application of a pulling force to an injured or diseased part of the body or an extremity while countertraction pulls in the opposite direction. • Two most common types are skin and skeletal traction. • One of the most common types of traction is Buck's traction.

. . . .

Definition: Chronic, systemic, progressive deterioration of connective tissue (synovium) of the joints; characterized by inflammation. Joint involvement is bilateral and symmetrical. In the joint, the normal cartilage becomes soft, fissures and pitting occur, and the cartilage thins. Spurs form and inflammation sets in. Severe cases may require joint replacement.
Causes: Classified as an immune complex disorder.
Assessment Findings: Fatigue; generalized weakness; anorexia; morning stiffness; joint deformity; bilateral inflammation of joints with the following symptoms: decreased ROM, joint pain, warmth, edema, erythema.
Treatment/Nursing Interventions: Corticosteroids, splinting, rest for joint deformity, immobilization, NSAIDs; utilize moist heat (warm, moist compress, whirlpool baths, hot showers in the morning); provide periods of rest; emphasize proper joint position; encourage assistive devices (elevated toilet seat, shower chair, walker, cane, wheelchair).

. . . .

TRACTION: GENERAL NURSING CARE

. . . .

TRACTION, SKELETAL

. . . .

TRACTION, SKIN

1. Ensure that all the ropes, weights, and pulleys are hanging freely.

2. Keep all lines off the traction ropes.

3. Do not lift the weights for any reason.

4. Avoid jarring the bed or equipment.

5. Complete frequent neuron checks.

6. Complete frequent circulatory checks, including color, temperature, pulses, and capillary refill.

7. Perform periodic skin assessments.

8. Keep the body in proper alignment.

9. Monitor for infection (fever, localized warmth, redness, swelling odor, or increased pain).

10. Do not massage the calves.

11. Increase fluid and fiber intake unless contraindicated.

12. Instruct the client to cough and deep breathe.

13. Encourage the client to utilize an overhead trapeze bar.

14. Provide diversionary activities.

. . . .

Definition: A form of traction that is applied mechanically to the bone with pins, wires, or tongs. In place for longer periods than skin traction, this method is used to align injured bones and joints or to treat joint contractures and congenital hip dysplasia. The long-term pull keeps the injured bones and joints aligned. The physician inserts a pin or wire into the bone, either partially or completely, to align and immobilize the injured body part. The amount of weight applied ranges from 5 to 45 pounds. **Nursing Care:** Monitor color, motion, and sensation of the affected extremity; monitor the insertion sites for redness, swelling, drainage, or increased pain; and provide insertion site care as ordered.

. . . .

Definition: A form of traction used for short-term treatment (48 to 72 hours) until skeletal traction or surgery is possible. Tape, boots, or splints are applied directly to the skin to maintain alignment, assist in reduction, and help decrease muscle spasms in the injured extremity. The traction weights are usually limited to 5 to 10 pounds. Cervical or pelvic skin traction may require heavier weights applied intermittently. The client should be positioned with the head of the bed elevated 30 to 40 degrees, and weights are attached to a pulley system over the head of the bed.

NCLEX-RN Flash Review

TRACTION, TYPES OF

Type	Description
Buck's (extension) Traction	• Used to alleviate muscle spasms and immobilize a lower limb by maintaining a straight pull on the limb with the use of weights. • A boot device/appliance attaches the traction. • Weights (limit 8 to 10 pounds) are attached to a pulley and hang freely over the edge of bed; elevation of the foot of bed is required.
Russell's (sling) Traction	• Skin traction composed of Buck's extension on the foreleg, three pulleys at the bottom, and a sling under the knee. • Affords more freedom of movement than Buck's.
Pelvic Skin Traction	• Utilized to relieve lower back, hip, or leg pain or to reduce muscle spasms. • A traction belt is applied snugly over the pelvis and iliac crest, and then the weights are attached.
Balanced Suspension Traction	• Utilized with skin or skeletal traction to approximate fractures of the femur, tibia, or fibula. • Counterforce other than the client is employed. • Client should be positioned in a low Fowler's position on either the side or the back, with a 20-degree angle from the thigh to the bed. • Protection of the skin from breakdown is imperative.
Dunlop's Traction	• Horizontal traction is used to align fractures of the humerus; vertical traction maintains the forearm in proper alignment. • Nursing care is the same as for Buck's traction.

• •

PART II

AGNOSIA

. . . .

ALEXIA

. . . .

APRAXIA

Definition: A neuropsychological disorder characterized by the inability to recognize common objects, persons, or sounds in the absence of perceptual disability. There are three major types of agnosia: visual agnosia, auditory agnosia, and tactile agnosia.

Causes: Lesions to the parietal and temporal lobes of the brain, regions involved in storing memories and associations of objects. The condition may arise following head trauma or stroke, or following carbon monoxide poisoning or anoxia.

. . . .

Definition: Loss of the ability to read.

. . . .

Definition: Inability to perform purposeful movements in the absence of motor problems.

AUTONOMIC DYSREFLEXIA

· ·

BABINSKI REFLEX

· ·

BELL'S PALSY

Definition: Syndrome characterized by paroxysmal hypertension, brady-cardia, excessive sweating, facial flushing, nasal congestion, pilomotor responses, and headache. Also known as hyperreflexia. The syndrome occurs with spiral lesions above T6 after the period of spinal shock is complete.
Causes: Triggers include visceral stimulation from a distended bladder or impacted rectum. The syndrome is a neurological emergency and must be treated immediately to prevent the development of a hypertensive stroke.
Treatment/Nursing Interventions: Priority interventions include raising the head of the bed; loosening tight clothing; checking for bladder distention, kinked urinary catheter, fecal impaction, or other noxious stimulus; and administer antihypertensive medications as ordered.

• •

Definition: Dorsiflexion of the big toe with extension; elicited by firmly stroking the lateral aspect of the sole of the foot.

• •

Definition: Caused by a lower motor neuron lesion of the 7th cranial nerve. This nerve controls facial muscles on one side of the face, which becomes swollen. As a result, the face feels stiff and half of the face appears to droop, smile is one-sided, and the client's eye resists closing.
Causes: Infection, trauma, tumor, meningitis, hemorrhage.
Assessment Findings: Loss of taste; flaccid facial muscles; inability to raise eyebrow, frown, smile, close eyelids, or puff cheeks; upward movement of eyes when attempting to close the eyelids.
Treatment/Nursing Interventions: Apply facial sling to prevent stretching of weak muscles if ordered; encourage facial exercises to prevent loss of muscle tone; provide/promote frequent mouth care; instruct client to chew on unaffected side; protect the eyes from dryness and prevent injury.
Special Considerations: Recovery usually occurs in a few weeks, without residual effects.

BRUDINSKI REFLEX

. . . .

CALORIC TESTING

. . . .

CEREBRAL PERFUSION PRESSURE (CPP), CALCULATION OF

Definition: A sign of meningeal irritation. Involuntary flexion of the hip and knee when the neck is passively flexed.

• •

Definition: Test is performed at bedside by introducing cold water into the external auditory canal. If the eighth cranial nerve is stimulated, nystagmus rotates toward the irrigated ear. If no nystagmus occurs, a pathological condition is present.

• •

Definition: difference between the mean arterial pressure (MAP) and the intracranial pressure (ICP).

CPP = MAP – ICP

This represents the pressure gradient driving cerebral blood flow (CBF), and hence oxygen and metabolite delivery. The normal brain autoregulates its blood flow to provide a constant flow regardless of blood pressure by altering the resistance of cerebral blood vessels. These homeostatic mechanisms are often lost after head trauma (cerebral vascular resistance is usually increased), and the brain becomes susceptible to changes in blood pressure. Those areas of the brain that are ischemic, or at risk of ischemia, are critically dependent on adequate cerebral blood flow, and therefore cerebral perfusion pressure. Usual range is 60 to 100 mmHg.

CEREBRAL SPINAL FLUID, RECOGNITION/TESTING FOR

· ·

CRANIAL NERVES

· ·

CRANIOTOMY

Two ways to verify that cerebral spinal fluid (CSF) is leaking:
1. Test leaking fluid with a dextrostick. If it is positive for sugar, then it is CSF. (*Note:* If blood is present in fluid, then this is an unreliable way to check for CSF since blood has sugar.)
2. "Halo" or "ring" sign. Allow leaking fluid to drip onto a 4 × 4 gauze. Within a few minutes blood will run into the center. A yellowish ring will encircle the blood if CSF is present.

Number	Name	Function
I	Olfactory	Smell
II	Optic	Vision
III	Oculomotor	Upper eyelid elevation, papillary constriction, extraocular movement
IV	Trochlear	Downward and inward eye movement
V	Trigeminal	Corneal reflex, face and scalp sensation, chewing
VI	Abducens	Lateral eye movement
VII	Facial	Taste, expression in forehead, eye movement
VIII	Acoustic	Hearing and balance
IX	Glossopharyngeal	Taste, swallowing, salivation
X	Vagus	Gag reflex, swallowing, talking, sensation of the throat and larynx
XI	Spinal accessory	Head rotation, shoulder shrug
XII	Hypoglossal	Tongue movement

Definition: Surgical procedure that involves an incision through the cranium to remove an accumulation of blood or tumor.
Complications: Increased ICP from cerebral edema, hemorrhage, or obstruction of the normal blood flow. Other complications that may develop are hematomas, hypovolemic shock, hydrocephalus, respiratory and neurogenic complications, pulmonary edema, and wound infections. Specific concerns related to fluid and electrolyte imbalances include the development of diabetes insipidus and inappropriate secretion of antidiuretic hormone.
Treatment/Preparation: Assure that preoperative measures include a full explanation to the client and family, that informed consent has been obtained prior to the procedure, and that the client is prepared to have his or her head shaved (as ordered; usually completed in the operating room). Craniotomy preoperative medications may include corticosteroids to reduce swelling; agents and osmotic diuretics to reduce secretions, such as Atropine or Robinul; agents to reduce seizures, such as phenytoin; and prophylactic antibiotics.

NCLEX-RN Flash Review

CRANIOTOMY, POSTOPERATIVE CARE

. . . .

. . . .

DECORTICATE AND DECEREBRATE POSTURING

. . . .

DYSARTHRIA

Positioning after the procedure will differ related to the type of surgery (area) involved.

- Monitor vital signs every 30 to 60 minutes; assure proper postoperative positionng per physician's order.
- Observe for signs and symptoms of increased ICP.
- Monitor and intervene appropriately if there is a decrease in the client's level of consciousness, visual changes, aphasia, paralysis, or motor weakness.
- Maintain mechanical ventilation as ordered; maintain the head of the client in a midline neutral position while avoiding extreme hip or neck flexion.
- Monitor head dressing as ordered and mark drainage; notify physician if dressing becomes saturated with blood; monitor and measure output from drains; notify physician if more than 30–50 mL per shift.
- Maintain strict intake and outputs (I&O); maintain fluid restriction of 1,500 mL/day or as ordered.
- Monitor serum electrolyte levels.
- Apply ice packs or cool compresses as ordered and antiembolism stockings as ordered.
- Administer anticonvulsants, antacids, corticosteroids, and antibiotics as ordered, as well as analgesics as ordered for pain.

· ·

Decorticate (Flexor) Posturing: Flexure of one or both arms and possibly in legs; indicates damaged cortex.

Decerebrate (Extensor) Posturing: Stiff extension of one or both arms and possibly the legs; indicates a brain stem lesion.

· ·

Definition: Difficulty articulating.

DYSPHAGIA

. . . .

DYSPHASIA

. . . .

FLACCID POSTURING

Definition: Dysfunctional swallowing.

. . . .

Definition: Impairment of speech and verbal comprehension.

. . . .

Definition: No motor response display in any extremity.

GLASGOW COMA SCALE

. . . .

GUILLAIN-BARRÉ SYNDROME

. . . .

Variable	Response	Score*
Eye Opening	• Spontaneously • To verbal command • To pain • No response, even to painful stimuli	4 3 2 1

Motor Response	• To verbal command
	• To painful stimuli:
	  • Localizes pain
	  • Flexes/withdraws
	  • Flexor posturing (decorticate)
	  • Extensor posturing (decerebrate)
	  • No motor response to pain
		6
		
		5
		4
		3
		2
		1

Verbal Response	• Oriented and converses • Disoriented, converses • Uses inappropriate words • Incomprehensible sounds • No verbal response	5 4 3 2 1

*Highest possible score is 15 points; a score lower than 8 indicates coma.

• •

Definition: Clinical syndrome of unknown origin involving peripheral and cranial nerves.

Causes: Usually preceded by a respiratory infection 1 to 4 weeks prior to the onset. A small percentage of clients diagnosed with this syndrome are left with residual disability.

Assessment Findings: Paresthesia; muscle weakness of legs progressing to the upper extremities, trunk, and face; paralysis of the ocular, facial, and oropharyngeal muscles, causing marked difficulty in talking, chewing, and swallowing. Assess for breathlessness, shallow and irregular breathing, use of accessory muscles while breathing, any change in respiratory pattern, and paradoxic inward movement of the upper abdominal wall while in a supine position (indicating weakness and impending paralysis of the diaphragm). Increasing pulse rate and disturbances in rhythm, transient hypertension, orthostatic hypotension, possible pain in the back and in calves of legs, weakness or paralysis of the intercostal and diaphragm muscles; may develop quickly.

Treatment/Nursing Interventions: Monitor for respiratory distress and initiate intubation and mechanical ventilation as indicated. Treatment is based on client presentation.

Special Considerations: Constant monitoring of these clients is required to prevent life-threatening acute respiratory failure. Full recovery usually occurs within several months to a year after onset of symptoms.

• •

HEAD INJURY

....

**HEAD INJURY, CLIENT EDUCATION
DISCHARGE INSTRUCTIONS**

....

Definition: A trauma to the skull, resulting in mild to extensive damage to the brain. Immediate complications include cerebral bleeding, hematomas, infection, seizures, and uncontrolled increased ICP. Can be open, such as lacerations, or closed, such as concussion, fractures, and hematomas. The term *head trauma* is used primarily to signify craniocerebral trauma, which includes an alteration in consciousness, no matter how brief.

Causes: Motor vehicle accidents; falls; firearms; assaults; sports-related injuries.

Assessment Findings: Depends on the type of injury. Assessment findings result from an increased ICP. Changing neurological signs, vital signs, airway and breathing patterns, reflexes; headache, nausea, vomiting, visual disturbances, papillary changes, and papilledema; nuchal rigidity; CSF drainage from the ears or nose; seizure activity; posturing.

Treatment/Nursing Interventions: Maintain respiratory status and patent airway; monitor neurological status and vital signs for signs of increased ICP, pain, and restlessness; maintain head of bed elevation to reduce venous pressure; prevent neck flexion; initiate seizure precautions; assess cranial nerve function, reflexes, and motor sensory function; check for CSF drainage; monitor for drainage from the nose or ears (may be CSF); monitor for signs of infection; prevent complications of immobility; instruct the client to avoid coughing. Surgical intervention may include a craniotomy.

. . . .

1. Instruct the client's caregiver to arouse the client every 3 to 4 hours for the first 24 hours, or set an alarm clock.

2. Instruct the client to anticipate dizziness and headaches.

3. Instruct the client not to blow his or her nose; try to prevent sneezing.

4. Instruct the client to use acetaminophen for headaches.

5. Instruct the client not to exercise for 2 or 3 days following injury.

6. Instruct the client to contact the physician if any of the following occur: blurred vision or diplopia; poor coordination in walking or grasping; drainage (serous or bloody) from the nose (rhinorrhea) or ears (otorrhea); forceful vomiting; increased sleepiness; slurred speech; headache that does not respond to medication or continues to get worse; occurrence of a seizure.

. . . .

HEAD INJURY, TYPES OF, I

· ·

HEAD INJURY, TYPES OF, II

· ·

Type	Description
Concussion	A jarring of the brain within the skull, with no loss of consciousness. May affect memory, speech, reflexes, balance, and coordination. Transient, self-limiting.
Contusion	Bruising of the brain tissue. Causes multiple areas of petechial hemorrhages. Blood supply is altered in the area of injury; swelling, ischemia, and increased ICP may result. Assessment findings include headache, papillary changes, dizziness, unilateral weakness. May last several hours to weeks.
Skull Fracture	*Linear:* Break in continuity of bone without alteration of relationship of parts. Low-velocity injury is often the cause. *Depressed:* Inward indentation of skull. Caused by a powerful blow. *Simple:* Linear or depressed skull fracture without fragmentation or communicating lacerations. Caused by low to moderate impact. *Comminuted:* Multiple linear fractures with fragmentation of the bone into many pieces. Caused by direct, high-momentum impact. *Compound:* Depressed skull fracture and scalp laceration with communicating pathway to intracranial cavity. Caused by severe head injury.

Type	Description
Epidural Hematoma	Neurological emergency. Hematoma forms between the dura and the skull from a tear in the meningeal artery or vein. A hematoma quickly forms, leading to an increased ICP. Often associated with temporary loss of consciousness, followed by a lucid period, which rapidly progresses to coma. Tentorial herniation may occur without immediate intervention.
Subdural Hematoma	A collection of blood between the dura and arachnoid area filling the brain vault; usually the result of a serious head injury. Can be *acute* (occurs in 24 to 48 hours after injury; immediate neurological deterioration of the client is noted; treatment involves craniotomy, and evacuation and decompression); *subacute* (occurs within 48 hours or 2 weeks after injury; alteration in mental status as hematoma develops; progression depends on size and location of hematoma; treatment involves evacuation and decompression); *chronic* (occurs weeks, months, usually ≥20 days post-injury). Often initial injury is forgotten by client. Nonspecific symptoms, does progress to altered LOC; evacuation and decompression may be completed; treatment may also include diuretics and anticonvulsants.
Intracerebral Hemorrhage	Multiple hemorrhages occur around a contused area.
Subarachnoid Hemorrhage	Bleeding occurs directly into the brain, ventricles, or subarachnoid space.

HEMIANOPSIA

· ·

HOMONYMOUS HEMIANOPSIA

· ·

INCREASED INTRACRANIAL PRESSURE (ICP)

PART II

Definition: Blindness in half the visual field.

· ·

Definition: Loss of half of the field of view on the same side in both eyes.

· ·

Definition: Life-threatening situation that results from an increase in any or all of the three components (brain tissue, blood, cerebral spinal fluid [CSF]) within the skull. Normal ICP ranges from 0 to 15 mmHg.
Causes: Cerebral edema caused by blunt trauma; fluid and electrolyte imbalances; brain tumors; intracranial hemorrhage caused by epidural or subdural bleeding; subarachnoid hemorrhage, hydrocephalus; cerebral embolism or thrombosis.
Assessment Findings: *Early:* Restlessness, irritability, lethargy. *Intermediate:* Unequal pupil responses, projectile vomiting, vital sign changes. *Late:* Decreased level of consciousness, decreased reflexes, hypoventilation, dilated pupils, posturing.
Treatment/Nursing Interventions: Elevation of the head of bed 30 degrees with head in the neutral position; intubation and mechanical ventilation; ICP monitoring; cerebral oxygen monitoring; maintenance of PaO_2 at 100 mmHg or greater; maintenance of fluid balance and assessment of osmolality; maintenance of systolic arterial pressure 100 to 160 mmHg; maintenance of cerebral perfusion pressure (CPP) ≥60mmHg, reduction of cerebral metabolism (e.g., high-dose barbiturates). Medication therapy includes osmotic diuretics (Mannitol); antiseizure medications (e.g., phenytoin [Dilantin]); corticosteroids (dexamethasone [Decadron] for brain tumors, bacterial meningitis); histamine (H_2)-receptor antagonist (e.g., cimetidine [Tagament]) or proton pump inhibitor (e.g., pantoprazole [Protonix]) to prevent GI ulcers and bleeding.

KERNIG'S SIGN

· ·

MEAN ARTERIAL PRESSURE (MAP), CALCULATION FOR

· ·

MENINGEAL IRRITATION, SIGNS AND SYMPTOMS OF

Definition: Loss of the ability of a supine client to straighten the leg completely when it is fully flexed at the knee and hip; client will experience pain. Indicates meningeal irritation.

. . . .

$$\frac{(2 \times Diastolic) + Systolic}{3}$$

Diastole counts twice as much as systole because $\frac{2}{3}$ of the cardiac cycle is spent in diastole. A MAP of about 60 is necessary to perfuse coronary arteries, brain, and kidneys. Usual range: 70 to 110.

. . . .

General Findings
Irritability
Nuchal rigidity
Severe, constant headache
Generalized muscle aches and pains
Tachycardia
Fever and chills
Nausea and vomiting
Nystagmus
Photophobia
Abnormal pupil response and eye movement
Brudzinski's sign
Kerning's sign
Motor response: Hemiparesis, hemiplegia, and decreased muscle tone Cranial nerve dysfunction III, IV, VI, VII, and VIII
Memory changes: Short attention span; bewilderment; personality and behavioral changes

MENINGITIS

....

MULTIPLE SCLEROSIS (MS)

....

Definition: An inflammation of the arachnoid and pia mater of the brain and spinal cord.

Causes: Caused by bacterial and viral organisms (fungal and protozol meningitis can occur). Cerebrospinal fluid is analyzed to determine which type is present. Transmission occurs in areas of high population density and in crowded living areas. Transmission of meningitis is by direct contact, including droplets. Predisposing factors include: skull fracture, brain or spinal surgery, use of nasal sprays, upper respiratory or sinus infections, or compromised immune system.

Assessment Findings: General signs of meningeal irritation; red macular rash with meningococcal meningitis; abdominal and chest pain with viral meningitis.

Treatment/Nursing Interventions: Monitor vital and neurological signs; assess for signs of increased ICP; perform cranial nerve assessment; monitor for seizure activity; maintain isolation precautions as indicated for bacterial meningitis; assure urine and stool precautions with viral meningitis; elevate the head of the bed 30 degrees while avoiding neck and extreme hip flexion; administer analgesics and antibiotics as ordered.

· ·

Definition: Believed to be autoimmune in origin. Demyelinating disease resulting in the destruction of CNS myelin and consequent disruption in the transmission of nerve impulses. Diagnosis determined by a combination of data: presenting symptoms, increased white matter density seen on CAT scan, presence of plaque seen on MRI, CSF electrophoresis shows presence of oligoclonal (IgG) bands.

Causes: Unknown. Thought to be a complicated interaction of the immune system, environment, infectious disease, and genetics.

Assessment Findings: Optic neuritis, scotomas, speech impairment, swallowing difficulties, impaired bladder and bowel function, unusual fatigue, weakness and clumsiness, gait disturbances, intention tremors, and numbness on one side of the face.

Treatment/Nursing Interventions: Orient client to the environment and teach strategies to maximize vision, initiate a voiding schedule, and encourage adequate fluid intake, high-fiber foods, and a bowel regimen for constipation; administer steroid therapy and chemotherapeutic medications in acute exacerbations to shorten length of attack. Medication therapy may include ACTH, cortisone, Cytoxan, and other immunosuppressive medications. Teach client about infection prevention.

Special Considerations: Symptoms involving motor function usually begin in the upper extremities, with weakness progressing to spastic paralysis. Bowel and bladder dysfunction occurs in 90% of cases. More common in women.

· ·

MYASTHENIA GRAVIS

. . . .

NUCHAL RIGIDITY

. . . .

OCULOCEPHALIC REFLEX (DOLL'S EYE REFLEX)

Definition: Disorder affecting the neuromuscular transmission of impulses in the voluntary muscles of the body. Considered an autoimmune disease characterized by the presence of acetylcholine receptor antibodies (AChRs), which interfere with neuronal transmission.

Causes: The exact cause is unknown. In some cases, it may be associated with tumors of the thymus.

Assessment Findings: Diplopia; ptosis; masklike affect; weakness of laryngeal and pharyngeal muscles (dysphagia, choking, food aspiration, difficulty speaking); muscle weakness improved by rest, worsened by activity. Clients may experience a myasthenic crisis (attributed to disease worsening; may result in respiratory failure) associated with undermedication, or a cholinergic crisis (attributed to anticholinesterase overdosage; symptoms include diaphoresis, diarrhea, and fasciculations).

Treatment/Nursing Interventions: Tracheostomy kit at bedside (treatment of myasthenic crisis), schedule nursing activities to conserve energy; instruct client to avoid situations that create fatigue or physical or emotional stress; bed rest may be implemented; teach strategies to avoid bladder and respiratory infection; encourage coughing and deep breathing exercises every 4 to 6 hours; administer cholinergic medications (pyridostigmine bromide [Mestinon]).

Special Considerations: Usually affects females between the ages of 10 and 40 and males over age 60. Advanced cases may experience respiratory failure, bladder and bowel incontinence.

· ·

Definition: Stiff neck; flexion of the neck onto the chest causes intense pain. A sign of meningeal irritation.

· ·

Definition: When normal, the client's head is moved from side to side: the eyes look in the direction opposite that of the turning. In contrast, when abnormal, the client's eyes remain in a fixed, midline position when the head is turned from side to side (possible brainstem involvement). Contraindicated until the risk of spinal cord injury is ruled out.

PARKINSON'S DISEASE

· ·

RESPIRATORY PATTERNS, ABNORMAL

· ·

Definition: A degenerative disease caused by the depletion of dopamine, which interferes with the inhibition of excitatory impulses, resulting in a dysfunction of the extrapyramidal system. It is slow and progressive, resulting in a crippling disability.

Causes: Exact causes are unknown; however, it is believed to be linked to genetic and environmental factors.

Assessment Findings: Rigidity of extremities; masklike facial expressions with associated difficulty in chewing, swallowing, and speaking; drooling; emotional lability; stooped posture and slow, shuffling gait; tremors at rest, "pill rolling" movement.

Treatment/Nursing Interventions: Schedule activities later in the day, instruct client not to rush self-care activities; encourage rest periods between activities; instruct client to utilize a walker or cane; encourage client to speak slowly and clearly; provide a soft diet if client has difficulty swallowing; administer antiparkinsonian medications as ordered.

Special Considerations: Debilitation can result in falls, self-care deficits, failure of body systems, and depression. Interventions are directed to providing safety measures. In this disorder the pathophysiology involves an imbalance between acetylcholine and dopamine, so symptoms are often controlled by administering a dopamine precursor such as levodopa (Dopar).

Type	Description
Cheyne-Stokes	Rhythmic respirations, with periods of apnea; can indicate a metabolic dysfunction, or dysfunction in the cerebral hemisphere or basal ganglia.
Neurogenic Hyperventilation	Regular rapid and deep sustained respirations; indicates a dysfunction in the low midbrain and middle pons.
Apneustic	Irregular respirations, with pauses at the end of inspiration and expiration; indicates a dysfunction in the middle or caudal pons.
Ataxic	Totally irregular in rhythm and depth; indicates dysfunction in the medulla.
Cluster	Cluster of breaths with irregularly spaced pauses; indicates a dysfunction in the medulla and pons.

SEIZURE

PART
II

. . . .

SEIZURE, TYPES OF: GENERALIZED SEIZURES, I

. . . .

Definition: An abnormal, sudden, excessive discharge of electrical activity within the brain.

Causes: Genetic factors; infection; tumors; trauma; toxicity; metabolic or circulatory disorders.

Assessment Findings: Seizure history: occurrences before, during, and after the seizure; loss of motor activity or bowel and bladder function or loss of consciousness during the seizure; aura: sensation that warns the client of an impending seizure; prodromal signs: mood changes, insomnia, and irritability; occurrences during the postictal state: sleepiness, headache, loss of consciousness, and impaired speech or thinking.

Treatment/Nursing Interventions: Support the ABCs; note the time and duration of seizure activity; apply oxygen; prepare for suctioning; if client is standing or sitting, place the client on the floor and protect the head; turn the client to the side to allow secretions to drain while maintaining airway; monitor for urination. Administer antiseizure medications as ordered; for tonic-clonic seizures: phenytoin (Dilantin), carbamazepine (Tegretol), phenobarbital (Luminal), and fosphenytoin (Cerebyx); for absent seizures: ethosuximide (Zarontin), valporic acid (Depakene). Pad side rails; monitor serum drug levels; tape oral airway to the head of the bed; encourage the client to wear a Medic-Alert bracelet.

Special Considerations: Epilepsy is a disorder characterized by chronic seizure activity and indications of central nervous system or brain irritation. If a client is having a seizure, maintain a patent airway. Do NOT force the jaw open or place anything in the client's mouth. Medication noncompliance is the most common case of increased seizure activity.

Type	Description
Tonic-Clonic	May begin with an aura. The tonic phase involves the stiffening or rigidity of the muscles of the arms and legs and lasts about 10 to 20 seconds, followed by a loss of consciousness. The clonic phase involves hyperventilation and jerking of the extremities and lasts about 30 seconds. Full recovery from the seizure may take several hours.
Absence	A seizure that lasts for seconds, and the client may or may not lose consciousness. No loss or change in muscle tone is observed. Seizures may occur several times a day. The client may appear to be daydreaming. This type of seizure is common in children.
Myolonic	Present as a brief generalized jerking or stiffening of extremities. The client may collapse to the ground from the seizure
Atonic or Akinetic (Drop Attacks)	Sudden momentary loss of muscle tone. The client may drop to the ground as a result of the seizure.

SEIZURE, TYPES OF: GENERALIZED SEIZURES, II

....

SPINAL CORD INJURY (SCI)

....

Type	Description
Simple Partial	Produces sensory symptoms accompanied by motor symptoms that are localized or confined to a specific area. The client remains conscious and may also report having an aura.
Complex Partial	A psychomotor seizure. The area of the brain most commonly involved is the temporal lobe. The seizure is characterized by periods of altered behavior of which the client is unaware. The client loses consciousness for a few seconds.

Definition: Disruption in nervous system function, which may result in complete or incomplete loss of motor and sensory function. Changes occur in the function of all physiologic systems. Injury is described by the location of injury to the spinal cord. The most common sites are C5, C6, C7, T12, and L1 (physical assessment should concentrate on respiratory status, especially with injuries at C3 to C5, as the cervical plexus innervates the diaphragm). Damage can range from contusion to complete transaction. Permanent impairment cannot be determined until the edema of the spinal cord resolves, usually by 1 week.

Causes: Motor vehicle collisions, acts of violence, sports-related injuries, diseases (cancer, arthritis, osteoporosis, spinal tumors).

Assessment Findings: Dependent on the level of injury (based on the lowest spinal cord segment with intact motor and sensory function); respiratory status changes; motor and sensory changes below the level of injury; total sensory and motor paralysis below the level of injury; loss of reflexes below the level of injury; loss of bladder and bowel control; urinary retention and bladder distention; presence of sweat, which does not occur on paralyzed areas.

Treatment/Nursing Interventions: Emergency management is critical as improper movement can cause further damage and loss of neurological function; assess the respiratory pattern and maintain a patent airway; prevent head flexion, rotation, or extension; during immobilization, utilize proper handling techniques; in cervical injuries, skeletal traction is maintained by use of skull tongs or halo ring; high-dose corticosteroids are often given in the first 8 to 24 hours to control edema; evaluate for the presence of spinal shock or autonomic dysreflexia and treat appropriately; watch for paralytic ileus; suction with caution.

SPINAL CORD INJURY, SPECIFIC ASSESSMENT FINDINGS

. . . .

SPINAL SHOCK

. . . .

SPINAL SHOCK AND AUTONOMIC DYSREFLEXIA, DIFFERENCES BETWEEN

Type of Injury	Assessment Findings
Cervical-Level Injuries	Injuries to C2 to C3 are usually fatal; C4 is the major innervation to the diaphragm by the phrenic nerve; involvement above C4 causes respiratory difficulty and paralysis of all four extremities; clients can have movement in the shoulder if the injury is at C5 through C8, and may also have decreased respiratory reserve.
Thoracic-Level Injuries	Loss of movement of the chest, trunk, bowel, bladder, and legs can occur, depending on the level of injury; leg paralysis (paraplegia) may occur; autonomic dysreflexia with lesions or injuries above T6 and in the cervical lesions may occur; visceral distention from a noxious stimulus such as a distended bladder or an impacted rectum may cause reactions such as sweating, hypertension, bradycardia, nasal stuffiness, and gooseflesh.
Lumbar and Sacral-Level Injuries	Loss of movement and sensation of the lower extremities may occur; S2 and S3 center on micturation; therefore, below this level, the bladder will contract but not empty (neurogenic bladder); injury S2 in males allows them to have an erection, but they are unable to ejaculate because of sympathetic nerve damage; injury between S2 and S4 damages the sympathetic and parasympathetic response, preventing sexual function (erection and ejaculation).

Definition: Complete loss of all reflex, motor, sensory, and autonomic activity below the lesion of injury. This is a medical emergency that occurs immediately after the injury.

Assessment Findings: Hypotension, bradycardia, complete paralysis and lack of sensation below lesion, and bowel and bladder distension.

Treatment/Nursing Interventions: Imperative to reverse spinal shock as quickly as possible. Spinal cord compression lasting for 12 to 24 hours can result in permanent paralysis.

Spinal Shock	Flaccid paralysis; loss of reflex activity below the level of injury; bradycardia; paralytic ileus; hypotension
Autonomic Dysreflexia	Sudden onset, severe throbbing headache; severe hypertension; sweating; nausea; flushing above the level of the injury; nasal stuffiness; pale extremities below the level of the injury; dilated pupils or blurred vision; goose bumps; restlessness and feeling of apprehension

STROKE, MANIFESTATIONS OF

. . . .

STROKE OR CEREBRAL VASCULAR ACCIDENT (CVA)

. . . .

TETRAPLEGIA AND PARAPLEGIA

Right-Brain Damage	• Paralyzed left side: hemiplegia; left-sided neglect; spatial-perceptual deficits; tendency to deny or minimize problems; rapid performance, short attention span; impulsive, safety problems; impaired judgment; impaired time concepts.
Left-Brain Damage	• Paralyzed right side: hemiplegia; impaired speech/language aphasias; impaired right/left discrimination; slow performance, caution; awareness of deficits: depression, anxiety; impaired incomprehension related to language, math.

Definition: Sudden loss of brain function resulting from a disruption in the blood supply to a part of the brain. Classified as ichemic or hemorrhagic. Central nervous system (CNS) involvement related to the cause of CVA: Hemorrhagic type is caused by a slow or fast hemorrhage into the brain tissue. Ischemic type is caused by a clot lodged in one of the arteries of the brain blocking the blood supply.

Causes: Hypertension; previous transient ischemic attacks (TIAs); cardiac disease (atherosclerosis, valve disease, history of arrhythmias, particularly atrial flutter or atrial fibrillation), advanced age, diabetes, oral contraceptives; smoking.

Assessment Findings: Presenting symptoms are related to specific areas of brain affected. *General findings:* motor loss, usually exhibited as a hemiparesis or hemiplegia; communication loss, exhibited as dysarthria, dysphasia, aphasia, or apraxia; perceptual disturbance that can be visual, spatial, and sensory; impaired mental acuity or psychological changes, such as decreased attention span, memory loss, depression, lability, and hostility; incontinence or retention.

Treatment/Nursing Interventions: Control of hypertension; maintain proper body alignment while client is in bed; position client to minimize edema, prevent contractures, and maintain skin integrity; perform range of motion (ROM); encourage to participate in activities of daily living (ADLs) as able; analyze bladder elimination pattern, initiate speech therapy, teach client that modifications may include a soft diet (pureed foods, thickened liquids) and head positioning, encourage family members to join support groups.

Tetraplegia (Quadriplegia)	Injury occurring between C1 and C8; paralysis involving all four extremities.
Paraplegia	Injury occurring between T1 and L4; paralysis involving only the lower extremities.

BREAST CANCER

. . . .

BREAST SELF-EXAMINATION (BSE), INSTRUCTIONS FOR

. . . .

Definition: Classified as invasive when it penetrates tissues surrounding the mammary duct and grows in an irregular pattern. Diagnosis is made by breast biopsy through needle aspiration or by surgical removal of the tumor with microscopic examination for malignant cells.

Causes: Risk factors: Age, family history of breast cancer, early menarche and late menopause; previous cancer of the breast, uterus, or ovaries; obesity; high-dose exposure of radiation to the chest.

Assessment Findings: Asymmetry of breast, skin dimpling, flattening, and nipple deviation are suggestive of lesion, skin coloring and thickening, large pores, sometimes called *peau d'orange* (orange peel appearance), changes in the nipple; discharge from nipple; mass is painless, nontender, hard, irregular in shape, and nonmobile; majority of malignant lesions are found in the upper outer quadrant of the breast (tail of Spence).

Treatment/Nursing Interventions: Surgical interventions include modified radical mastectomy (most common), local excision (lumpectomy), radical mastectomy (less common), or breast reconstruction. Radiation, hormonal therapy, and chemotherapy are also utilized.

· ·

1. While in the shower or bath, when breasts are wet and slippery with soap, examine the breasts.

2. Utilize the pads of the second, third, and fourth fingers to press every part of the breasts firmly.

3. Use the right hand to examine the left breast, and the left hand to examine the right breast.

4. Using the pads of the fingers on the left hand, examine the entire right breast using small circular motions in a spiral or up-and-down motion so that the entire breast area is examined. Repeat the same procedure to examine the left breast.

5. Repeat the pattern of palpation under the arm.

6. Check for any lumps, hard knots, or thickening of tissue.

Note: Perform monthly 7 to 10 days after menses. Postmenopausal clients or clients who have had a hysterectomy should select a specific day of the month and perform BSE monthly on that day.

· ·

LUNG CANCER

. . . .

METASTASIS: COMMON SITES

. . . .

Definition: Tumor may represent the primary site or may be metastatic from a primary lesion elsewhere. There are two main types: small cell lung cancer (SCLC) and non–small cell lung cancer (NSCLC); epidermal (squamous cell), adenocarcinoma, and large cell anaplastic carcinoma are classified as NSCLC because of their similar responses to treatment. Diagnosis is made by chest X-ray study, CT scan or MRI, bronchoscopy, and sputum studies that demonstrate a positive cytological study for cancer cells.

Causes: Cigarette smoking, also exposure to passive tobacco smoke, exposure to environmental and occupational pollutants.

Assessment Findings: Wheezing, dyspnea, hoarseness, chest pain, hemoptysis-blood-tinged purulent sputum, weakness, anorexia, weight loss, hoarseness, and diminished or absent breath sounds.

Treatment/Nursing Interventions: Vary with the degree/extent of malignancy. Radiation may be utilized preoperatively to reduce tumor mass. Surgical interventions include lobectomy, pneumonectomy, and lung-conserving resection. Chemotherapy is also used.

Special Consideration: Treatment may involve all three therapies: radiation, chemotherapy, and surgery.

. . . .

Initial Site	Common Sites of Metastasis
Bladder Cancer	Lung, bone, liver, pelvic, retroperitoneal structures
Brain Tumors/Cancer	Central nervous system
Breast Cancer	Bone, lung, brain, liver
Colorectal Cancer	Liver
Lung Cancer	Brain, liver
Prostate Cancer	Bone, spine, lung, liver, kidneys
Testicular Cancer	Lung, bone, liver, adrenal glands, retroperitoneal nodes

. . . .

TESTICULAR CANCER

PART
II

. . . .

**TESTICULAR SELF-EXAMINATION,
INSTRUCTIONS FOR**

. . . .

Definition: Tumors are often malignant and often metastasize quickly. They arise from germinal epithelium from the sperm-producing germ cells or from nongerminal epithelium from other structures in the testicles.

Causes: Generally unknown, but history of undescended testicles and genetic predisposition have been associated with testicular tumor development.

Assessment Findings: Painless testicular swelling occurs, dragging or pulling sensation in the scrotum, palpable lymphadenopathy, abdominal masses, and gynecomatia (may indicate metastasis), back, bone pain, or respiratory distress (late signs).

Treatment/Nursing Interventions: Surgical interventions includes orchiectomy (performed as soon as possible), retroperitoneal lymph node dissection (if lymph involvement). Medical interventions include postoperative irradiation to the lymphatic drainage pathways and multiple chemotherapy medications.

Special Considerations: Early recognition through self testicular examination is key.

. . . .

Step 1: Examine using a mirror. Using a mirror, examine the scrotum, looking for any lumps on the skin or swellings inside.

Step 2: Feel for differences between the testicles. Cradle the whole scrotum and testicles in the palm of the hand and feel for any differences between the testicles. One is usually larger and lying lower, and this is normal.

Step 3: Check for lumps and swellings. Use both hands and gently roll each testicle between thumb and forefinger, checking for any lumps or swellings. Be aware of heaviness or hardness in part or all of the testicle. The testicles should be smooth to touch except for the epididymis, which is a soft sausagelike tube that lies at the top and back of the testicles and carries sperm to the penis.

Note: Best time to completed exam is after a shower. Complete every month.

. . . .

ARTERIAL STEAL SYNDROME

. . . .

AZOTEMIA

. . . .

CONTINUOUS RENAL REPLACEMENT THERAPY (CRRT)

Definition: A syndrome that may develop following the insertion of an arteriovenous fistula when too much blood is diverted to the vein and arterial perfusion to the hand is compromised. Symptoms include hand pain; diminished/altered sensation; pale, cold hand; diminished or absent radial pulse; and poor capillary filling.

. . . .

Definition: The retention of nitrogenous waste products in the blood. It is a condition in which the patient's blood contains uncommon levels of urea, creatinine, and other compounds rich in nitrogen, and it is also one clinical characteristic of a wider condition known as uremia, which includes other conditions such as acidosis, anemia, hyperkalemia, hypertension, and hypocalcemia. The underlying cause is typically the kidneys' insufficient filtering of the blood. Direct causes may include certain antiviral medications, congestive heart failure, extended diarrhea or vomiting, kidney trauma, liver failure, severe burns, or shock.

. . . .

Definition: An alternative measure for treating acute renal failure. The uremic toxins are removed slowly and continuously. This allows for constant maintenance of acid-base and electrolyte balance in an unstable client. Types include:

CVVH = Continuous venovenous hemofiltration

CAVH = Continuous arteriovenous hemofiltration

CVVHD = Continuous venovenous hemodialysis

CAVHD = Continuous arteriovenous hemodialysis

SCUF = Slow continuous ultrafiltration

NCLEX-RN Flash Review

CREATININE CLEARANCE TEST

. . . .

CYSTITIS

. . . .

DIALYSIS, VASCULAR ACCESS FOR

Definition: A test that evaluates how well the kidneys remove creatinine from the blood. The test requires a blood sample and timed urine specimens. The urine specimen is usually collected for 24 hours, and the blood sample is drawn after the urine collection is completed. The test provides the best estimate of the glomerular filtration rate (GFR). The normal GFR is 125 mL/minute.

· ·

Definition: A urinary tract infection causing inflammation of the bladder from an infection, obstruction of the urethra, or other irritants.
Causes (not all-inclusive): Allergens or irritants (soaps, bubble bath, perfumed sanitary napkins), bladder distention, calculus, hormonal changes, indwelling catheters, sexual intercourse, urinary stasis, and loss of bacterial properties of prostatic secretions in males.
Assessment Findings: Frequency and urgency; burning on urination; inability to void; voiding small amounts of urine; hematuria; cloudy, dark, foul-smelling urine; abdominal and back pain; malaise; chills; fever; nausea and emesis; white blood cell count greater than 100,000 cells/mm^3 on urinalysis.
Treatment/Nursing Interventions: Obtain urine specimen for culture and sensitivity prior to administering prescribed antibiotics, increase fluid intake (3,000 mL/day), administer prescribed medications (may include analgesics, urinary antiseptics, antispasmodics, antibiotics, or antimicrobials), sitz baths and heat to abdomen as needed, proper care of indwelling urinary catheter, and avoidance of caffeine products and alcohol.
Special Considerations: Sexually active and pregnant women are most vulnerable to cystitis. Instruct client to take all medications as prescribed (complete entire course of antibiotics), have a urine culture completed following treatment, and follow the measures to prevent reoccurrence.

· ·

Fistula	A fistula uses the client's own tissue to connect an artery and vein, usually in the forearm.
Graft	A graft connects an artery to a vein using a piece of synthetic tubing. Grafts take less time to develop, so they can sometimes be used earlier for dialysis, but dialysis grafts may be subject to more clotting and infection rates than dialysis fistulas.
Peritoneal Catheter	Usually a plastic catheter is surgically implanted to allow the dialysis cleansing fluid (dialysate) to enter and leave the peritoneal cavity. In peritoneal dialysis, there is no direct connection to the bloodstream.
Temporary Dialysis Catheter	A short-term solution for emergency dialysis or while waiting for a dialysis fistula or graft to be ready. These are temporary central venous catheters (CVCs), which are plastic tubes or catheters placed into the main vein in the neck or chest.

DIET, ACID-ASH

PART II

· ·

DIET, ALKALINE-ASH

· ·

DIET, FOOD SOURCES HIGH IN PURINE, CALCIUM, AND OXALATE

Foods to Include
Meat, fish, oysters, poultry
Bread, cereal, whole grains
Cheese, eggs
Cranberries, prunes, plums, tomatoes
Corn and legumes

Outcome: Diet decreases the pH of urine and makes the urine more acidic.

· ·

Foods to Include
Fruits except cranberries, tomatoes, prunes, and plums
Rhubarb
Milk
Most vegetables
Small amounts of trout, beef, salmon, veal, and halibut

Outcome: Diet increases the urine pH and reduces the acidity of urine.

· ·

Purine*	High: Sardines, herring, mussels, liver, kidney, goose, venison, meat soups, sweetbreads Moderate: Chicken, salmon, crab, veal, mutton, bacon, pork, beef, ham
Calcium	High: Milk, cheese, ice cream, yogurt, sauces containing milk; all beans (except green beans), lentils; fish with fine bones (e.g., sardines, kippers, herring, salmon); dried fruits, nuts; Ovaltine, chocolate, cocoa
Oxalate	High: Dark roughage, spinach, rhubarb, asparagus, cabbage, tomatoes, beets, nuts, celery, parsley, runner beans; chocolate, cocoa, instant coffee, Ovaltine, tea; Worcestershire sauce

*Uric acid is a waste product from purine foods.

GLOMERULAR FILTRATION RATE (GFR)

. . . .

GLOMERULONEPHRITIS

. . . .

HEMODIALYSIS

Definition: The flow rate of filtered fluid through the kidney, an indicator of renal function.

· ·

Definition: A group of diseases that damage the glomeruli of the kidneys, commonly caused by an immunological reaction. Inflammation of the glomeruli results from an antigen-antibody reaction produced from an infection or autoimmune process elsewhere in the body. Results in loss of kidney function. Can be acute or chronic in nature; the acute form occurs 5 to 12 days following a streptococcal infection; the chronic form occurs after the acute phase or slowly over time.

Causes: Immunological or autoimmune diseases, history of pharyngitis or tonsillitis 2 to 3 weeks after symptoms, group A beta-hemolytic streptococcal infection.

Assessment Findings: *Acute:* Proteinuria, asymptomatic, hematuria, tea or cola-colored urine (due to hematuria), facial or periorbital edema, oliguria, hypertension, azotemia. *Chronic:* Symptoms of progressive renal failure.

Treatment/Nursing Interventions: Diuretics, antihypertensive medications, antibiotics, plasmapheresis; decrease sodium intake, protein restriction if azotemia is present, decrease foods in potassium, and fluid restriction.

Special Considerations: Complications include chronic renal failure, pulmonary edema, congestive heart failure, and hypertensive episodes.

· ·

Definition: Circulation of the client's blood through a compartment that contains an artificial semipermeable membrane surrounded by dialysate fluid, which removes excess body fluid by creating a pressure differential between the blood and the dialysate solution.

HEMODIALYSIS, COMPLICATIONS OF

. . . .

PERITONEAL DIALYSIS

. . . .

PERITONEAL DIALYSIS, COMPLICATIONS OF

Air embolus
Disequilibrium syndrome
Electrolyte alterations
Encephalopathy
Hemorrhage
Hepatitis
Hypotension
Sepsis
Shock

. . . .

Definition: Utilization of the peritoneal cavity and the peritoneum as the semipermeable membrane that removes excess fluid; a way to remove waste products from the blood when the kidneys can no longer do the job adequately. During the procedure, blood vessels in the abdominal lining (peritoneum) fill in for the kidneys, with the help of a fluid (dialysate) that flows into and out of the peritoneal space.

Differs from hemodialysis, a more commonly used blood-filtering procedure, in that treatments can occur in the home, at work, or while traveling. Not an option for everyone with kidney failure: clients must have manual dexterity (or a reliable caregiver) and the ability to care for themselves at home.

. . . .

Abdominal pain
Bladder or bowel perforation
Insufficient outflow
Leakage around the catheter site
Peritonitis

PERITONEAL DIALYSIS, CONTINUOUS AMBULATORY

. . . .

PYELONEPHRITIS

. . . .

RENAL FAILURE, ACUTE (ARF)

Definition: The dialysate is infused into the abdomen and remains there for a specific time period (2 to 6 hours). The dialysate is removed by gravity drainage after the scheduled period of time.

. . . .

Definition: A type of urinary tract infection that involves inflammation of the renal pelvis; can be acute or chronic in nature.

Causes: In acute form, often occurs following an invasive procedure of the urinary tract, or is due to the introduction of bacteria into the urethra. It develops a new infection or recurs as a relapse of a previous infection (can progress to bacteremia or chronic pyelonephritis). In chronic form, commonly occurs following chronic urinary flow obstruction with reflux and can lead to renal failure.

Assessment Findings: *Acute:* Nausea, fever, chills, dysuria, headache, flank pain on the affected side, frequency and urgency, costovertebral angle tenderness, cloudy, bloody, or foul-smelling urine. *Chronic:* Proteinuria, azotemia, poor urine concentrating ability.

Treatment/Nursing Interventions: Monitor for elevated temperature, evaluate vital signs, increase fluid intake to 3,000 mL/day, monitor urinary output (1,500 mL/24 hours), complete daily weight, and provide frequent rest periods. Advocate a high-calorie, low-protein diet; administer medications as prescribed (analgesics, antipyretics, antibiotics, urinary antiseptics, and antiemetics); and monitor for signs of renal failure.

Special Consideration: Chronic form is often diagnosed accidentally when the client is being evaluated for hypertension.

. . . .

Definition: The sudden loss of kidney function caused by renal cell damage from ischemic or toxic substances. It occurs abruptly and is reversible. It leads to hypoperfusion, cell death, and decomposition in renal function. The prognosis depends on the cause and condition of the client. Near-normal kidney function may resume gradually. The most common cause is hypotension and prerenal hypovolemia or exposure to a nephrotoxin.

RENAL FAILURE, ACUTE, CAUSES OF

· ·

RENAL FAILURE, ACUTE, CLINICAL MANIFESTATIONS OF

· ·

Prerenal	Factors external to the kidneys that reduce renal blood flow and lead to decreased glomerular perfusion and filtration. Caused by intravascular volume depletion, dehydration, decreased cardiac output, decreased peripheral vascular resistance, decreased renovascular blood flow, and prerenal obstruction or infection.
Intrarenal	Conditions that cause direct damage to the renal tissue (parenchyma), resulting in impaired nephron function. Caused by tubular necrosis, prolonged prerenal ischemia, intrarenal infection or obstruction, and nephrotoxicity (e.g., aminoglycoside antibiotics, contrast media)
Postrenal	Involves mechanical obstruction of urinary output. As the urine flow is obstructed, urine refluxes into the renal pelvis, impairing kidney function. Caused by benign prostatic hyperplasia, prostate cancer, calculi, trauma, and extrarenal tumors.

Urinary	• Decreased urinary output (oliguric, less than 400 mL/day; in older clients, may be 600–700 mL/day). • Internal and postrenal failure: fixed gravity, increased sodium in the urine, proteinuria, with glomerular membrane alteration, muddy brown casts. • Prerenal failure: past history of precipitating event; urine specific gravity may be high; high urinary sodium concentration and proteinuria. • High output failure: the kidney no longer filters urine; high urinary output, but the urine is dilute and does not contain waste products from filtering.
Cardiovascular	Pericarditis, pericardial effusion, arrhythmias caused by acidosis or hyperkalemia, congestive heart failure, hypotension followed by hypertension.
Respiratory	Pulmonary edema related to fluid overload, Kussmaul respirations due to metabolic acidosis, pleural effusions.
Hematological	Anemia, leukocytosis, altered platelet function leading to bleeding tendencies.
Neurological	Seizures, altered mentation, memory impairment, lethargy.
Fluid and Electrolyte Imbalances	Fluid retention, hyperkalemia, hyponatremia, metabolic acidosis.

RENAL FAILURE, ACUTE, MANAGEMENT OF

Medical Management	• Identify and treat precipitating causes of ARF. • Diuretic therapy and fluid challenges may be initiated. • Sorbitol (osmotic cathartic) may be administered with exchange resins to induce diarrhea to eliminate potassium ions. • Sodium polystyrene sulfonate (kayexalate), a cation-exchange resin, given by mouth or retention enema to remove potassium from the body. • Metabolic acidosis can be treated with IV sodium bicarbonate. • IV dopamine may be administered to enhance renal perfusion.
Dietary Management	• Fluid restriction; monitor intake and output; monitor serum plasma levels to regulate the intake of protein, potassium, and sodium; and increase intake of carbohydrates and protein of high biological value.
Dialysis Management	• Indications: volume overload, BUN level greater than 120 mg/dL, metabolic acidosis, increased potassium with electrocardiographic changes, plural effusion, and cardiac tamponade.

RENAL FAILURE, ACUTE, PHASES OF

Onset Phase	Oliguric Phase	Diuretic Phase	Recovery (Convalescent) Phase
Begins with a precipitating event.	• Urinary output decreases to less than 400 mL per 24 hours. • Increase in blood urea nitrogen (BUN), creatinine, uric acid, potassium, and magnesium levels and the presence of metabolic acidosis. • Duration is 1 to 3 weeks; the longer the duration, the less favorable the recovery. • Nonoliguric renal failure: also referred to as high output failure; urine is dilute and renal disease present. • These clients usually recover more quickly and have fewer complications.	• Often has a sudden onset within 2 to 6 weeks after oliguric phase. Diuresis up to 10 L/day; urine is very dilute. • Hypovolemia and hypotension can occur due to massive fluid losses. • BUN level stops rising. Urine creatinine clearance stabilizes. • Client at risk for hypokalemia and hyponatremia • May last for 1 to 3 weeks.	• Begins when the GFR increases. May take up to 12 months for renal function to become stabilized. • Usually some permanent loss of renal function, but remaining function is sufficient to maintain a healthy life (older adults are less likely to experience a return of full kidney function). • Complications include secondary infection, which is the most common cause of death.

RENAL FAILURE, CHRONIC (CRF)

. . . .

RENAL FAILURE, CHRONIC, MANAGEMENT OF

PART II

. . . .

RENAL FAILURE, CHRONIC: STAGE 1, DIMINISHED RENAL RESERVE

Definition: Also referred to as chronic kidney disease, it involves progressive, irreversible loss of kidney function such that the kidneys are no longer able to maintain the body environment. It is defined as either the presence of kidney damage or a glomerular filtration rate (GFR) $\leq$60 mL/minute for 3 months or longer (normal GFR is about 125 mL/minute and is reflected by urine creatinine clearance measurements).

• •

Medical Management	• Reduce serum potassium levels. • Administer antihypertension medications. • Administer diuretics: thiazide and loop diuretics. • Treatment of anemia: erythropoietin (Epogen, Procrit, Aranesp). • Treatment of renal osteodystrophy: phosphate binders and supplemental vitamin D.
Dietary Management	• Dietary intervention to treat weight loss and both adipose and muscle tissue. • Protein restriction. • Fluid restriction (600–1000 mL); adjust according to urinary output and/or dialysis. • Sodium restriction.
Dialysis Management	• As indicated.
Renal Transplantation	• As indicated.

• •

Diminished Renal Reserve	• Normal BUN and serum creatinine levels. • No signs or symptoms. • Healthy kidney tissues compensate for diseased tissue. • GFR 60% to 89% of normal.

• •

RENAL FAILURE, CHRONIC: STAGE 2, RENAL INSUFFICIENCY

. . . .

RENAL FAILURE, CHRONIC: STAGE 3, END-STAGE RENAL FAILURE

. . . .

Renal Insufficiency	• GFR is 25% of normal. • Mild anemia. • BUN and serum creatinine levels are elevated (azotemia); decreased urinary creatinine clearance. • Headaches. • Impaired urine concentration leading to nocturia, then polyuria.

. . . .

GFR	• GFR less than 10% of normal. • Severe azotemia. • Hyperkalemia, hyperphosphatemia, hypernatremia. • Metabolic acidosis. • Altered renin-angiotension system. • Decreased erythropoietin production.
Urinary System	Specific gravity of urine fixed at 1.010; proteinuria, casts, pyuria, hematuria; oliguria eventually leads to anuria less than 100 mL/24 hour.
Endocrine System	Hyperparathyroidism, which causes hypocalcemia and hyperphosphatemia, resulting in demineralization of the bones (renal osteodystrophy).
Hematological System	Bleeding, anemia, and infection.
Cardiovascular System	Congestive heart failure, hypertension, atherosclerotic heart disease, uremic pericarditis, pericardial effusion.
Gastrointestinal (GI) System	Anorexia, nausea, vomiting, uremic fector, GI bleeding, peptic ulcer disease, gastritis.
Metabolic System	Hyperglycemia, hyperlipidemia, gout, hyponatremia, carbohydrate intolerance.
Neurological System	Headaches, seizures, sleep disturbances.
Musculoskeletal System	Renal osteodystrophy, tissue calcification.
Integumentary System	Ecchymosis, uremic frost, yellow/gray discoloration, pruritus.

. . . .

RISK FACTORS: INTRARENAL FAILURE (KIDNEY TISSUE DISEASE)

PART II

. . . .

RISK FACTORS: POSTRENAL FAILURE (OBSTRUCTIVE PROBLEMS)

. . . .

RISK FACTORS: PRERENAL FAILURE (RENAL ISCHEMIA)

Risk Factor	Signs and Symptoms
Acute Tubular Necrosis	Hemolytic blood transfusion reaction; nephritic chemicals (lead, mercury, carbon tetrachloride); nephrotoxic medications (streptomycin, aminoglycoside antibiotics, and amphotercin-B); radiology contrast material
Infections	Acute glomerulonephritis, pyelonephritis, CMV, candidiasis
Diseases That Precipitate Vascular Changes	Atherosclerosis, diabetes mellitus, hypertension

· ·

Urinary and renal calculi
Bladder cancer, neuromuscular disorders
Benign prostatic hypertrophy
Urethral strictures
Trauma resulting in obstruction

· ·

Risk Factor	Signs and Symptoms
Circulatory Volume Depletion	Hemorrhage, dehydration
Decreased Cardiac Output	Pump failure and/or congestive heart failure, especially in older adults
Decreased Peripheral Resistance	Septic shock, anaphylaxis, antihypertensive medications
Volume Shifts	Third spacing of fluid, gram-negative sepsis, hypoalbuminemia
Vascular Obstruction	Renal artery occlusion, dissection abdominal aneurysm

SPECIFIC GRAVITY

. . . .

URINARY/RENAL CALCULI

. . . .

Definition: A urine test that measures the ability of the kidneys to concentrate urine. Normal value is 1.016 to 1.022 (may vary depending on laboratory). An increased reading (more concentrated urine) occurs with insufficient fluid intake, decreased renal perfusion, or increased antidiuretic hormone (ADH). A decreased reading (less concentrated urine) occurs with increased fluid intake or diabetes insipidus; it may also indicate renal disease or the kidneys' inability to concentrate urine.

• •

Definition: Stone formation anywhere in the urinary tract; the most common location for stones is in the pelvis of the kidney. Stones may be located through radiography of the kidneys, ureters, and bladder; intravenous pyelography; CT scanning; and renal ultrasound. Common types of stones include calcium oxalate or phosphate stones, cystine stones, struvite stones, and uric acid stones.
Causes: Family history, infection, urinary stasis, immobility, dehydration, excessive diuretic usage (dehydration), hypercalcemia and hyperparathyroidism, diet high in calcium, vitamin D, protein, oxalate, purines, or alkali.
Assessment Findings: Sudden, sharp, severe abdominal or flank pain (renal or ureteral colic), nausea and vomiting, pallor, and diaphoresis during episodes of pain, fever, hematuria, oliguria, or anuria (suggests obstruction; treat immediately).
Treatment/Nursing Interventions: Monitor vital signs and intake and output; increase fluid intake to 3,000 mL/day (aids in passage of stones); assess for fever, chills, infection; initiate intravenous fluid administration as prescribed; administer pain medications as prescribed (morphine or Dilaudid/hydromorphone), strain all urine; if stone passes, send to laboratory for analysis.
Special Considerations: Complications include recurrent stone formation, infection, or renal failure. Dietary modifications are based on the type of stone present.

• •

URINARY/RENAL CALCULI, DIETARY AND MEDICAL MANAGEMENT OF

. . . .

URINARY/RENAL CALCULI, MAJOR CATEGORIES OF

. . . .

Stone Type	Dietary Management	Medication Management
Calcium Oxalate Stones	• Acid-ash diet. • Decrease foods high in calcium and avoid oxalate food sources.	• Allupurinol, pyridoxine (vitamin B_6)
Calcium Phosphate Stones	• Acid-ash diet. • Decrease foods high in calcium, phosphate, and vitamin D.	• Phosphates, thiazide diuretics, allupurinol (Zyloprim)
Cystine Stones	• Alkaline-ash diet. • Avoid eggs, cheese, milk, and meat.	• Antibiotics
Struvite Stones	• Acid-ash diet. • Decrease foods high in phosphate. • Increase fluid intake to 3L/day unless contraindicated.	• Antibiotics
Uric Acid Stones	• Alkaline-ash diet. • Decrease foods high in purine.	• Allupurinol

Calcium Stones	Most common type. Occur more often in men than in women, and usually appear between the ages of 20 and 30; recurrent. Calcium can combine with other substances, such as oxalate (the most common substance) and phosphate to form the stone. Oxalate is present in certain foods. Diseases of the small intestine increase the risk of forming calcium oxalate stones.
Cystine Stones	Can form in people who have cystinuria. This type of stone runs in families and affects both men and women.
Struvite Stones	Mostly found in women who have a urinary tract infection. These stones can grow very large and can block the kidney, ureter, or bladder.
Uric Acid Stones	More common in men than in women. Occurs with gout and chemotherapy.

NCLEX-RN Flash Review

URINARY SYSTEM: COMMON ABNORMALITIES ASSESSMENT I

PART II

. . . .

URINARY SYSTEM: COMMON ABNORMALITIES ASSESSMENT II

. . . .

Finding	Description	Possible Etiology and Significance
Anuria	Technically no urination (24-hour urine output ≤100 mL)	Acute renal failure, end-stage renal disease, bilateral ureteral obstruction
Chemical Cystitis	Painful or difficult urination	Use of spermicides (diaphragm), excessive douching
Dysuria	Painful or difficult urination	Sign of urinary tract infection (UTI) and interstitial cystitis and a variety of pathologic conditions
Enuresis	Involuntary nocturnal urinating	Symptomatic lower urinary tract disorder
Frequency	Increased incident of urinating	Acutely inflamed bladder, retention with overflow, excess fluid intake
Hematuria	Blood in the urine	Cancer of the genitourinary tract, blood dyscrasias, renal disease, UTI, stones in the kidney or ureter, medications (anticoagulants)
Incontinence	Inability to voluntarily control discharge of urine	Neurogenic bladder, bladder infection, injury to external sphincter

Finding	Description	Possible Etiology and Significance
Nocturia	Frequency of urine at night	Renal disease with impaired concentrating ability, bladder obstruction, heart failure, diabetes mellitus
Oliguria	Diminished amount of urine in a given time (24-hour urine output of 100–400 mL)	Severe dehydration, shock, transfusion reaction, kidney disease, end-stage renal disease
Polyuria	Large amount of urine in a given time	Diabetes mellitus, diabetes insipidus, chronic renal failure, diuretics, excessive fluid intake
Retention	Inability to urinate even though bladder contains excessive amounts of urine	Finding after pelvic surgery, childbirth, catheter removal, neurogenic bladder
Stress Incontinence	Involuntary urination with increased pressure (sneezing or coughing)	Weakness of sphincter control

URINARY TRACT INFECTION (UTI)

. . . .

Definition: Stasis of the urine in the bladder and reflux of urine back into the original reservoir are the primary causes of these infections. Some common microorganisms causing the infections include *Escherichia coli* (most common), *Enterococcus*, *Klebsiella*, and *Staphylococcus*. There are two types: upper and lower.

Upper: *Pyelonephritis* is an inflammation of the renal pelvis and the parenchyma of the kidney(s).

Lower: *Cystitis*, inflammation/infection of the bladder, and *urethritis*, which is inflammation of the urethra.

· ·

ACUTE RESPIRATORY DISTRESS SYNDROME (ARDS)

....

ASTHMA

....

Definition: A condition characterized by increased capillary permeability in the alveolar capillary membrane, resulting in fluid leaking into the interstitial spaces and the alveoli and a decrease in pulmonary compliance.

Causes: Sepsis, fluid overload, trauma, shock, burns, neurological injuries, aspiration, pneumonia, embolism, shock.

Assessment Findings: Tachycardia, tachypnea, dyspnea, increasing hypoxia not responsive to increased levels of fraction of inspired O_2 (FiO_2), refractory hypoxia.

Treatment/Nursing Interventions: Identify and treat the underlying cause, maintain oxygenation via high levels of concentration or endotracheal intubation and mechanical ventilation with positive end-expiratory pressure (PEEP), suction client as needed, obtain and evaluate arterial blood gas (ABG) results, restrict fluid intake as ordered, evaluate hemodynamic pressure monitoring values, and provide adequate nutritional support to meet the client's increased metabolic needs. Administer diuretics, anticoagulants, or corticosteroids as prescribed.

Special Considerations: Clients are treated in the intensive care unit. ABG levels identify respiratory acidosis. Chest X-ray shows bilateral interstitial and alveolar infiltrates.

. . . .

Definition: Chronic inflammatory disorder of the airways that causes varying degrees of obstruction in the airways. Marked by inflammation and hyperresponsiveness to a variety of stimuli or triggers. Causes recurrent episodes of wheezing, breathlessness, chest tightness, and coughing associated with airflow obstruction that may be resolved spontaneously; it is often reversible.

Causes: Environmental factors, physiological factors, medications, occupational exposures, and food additives.

Assessment Findings: Restlessness, wheezing or crackles, absent or decreased breath sounds, use of accessory muscles while breathing, tachypnea, hyperventilation, prolonged exhalation, cyanosis, decreased oxygen saturation.

Treatment/Nursing Interventions: Acute interventions: place in high Fowler's position; administer O_2 as ordered; stay with client to offer support and decrease anxiety; administer bronchodilators as prescribed; auscultate lungs before, during, and after treatment.

Special Consideration: Status asthmaticus is a severe, life-threatening attack that must be treated immediately.

. . . .

BREATH SOUNDS

· ·

Type/Location	Description
Bronchial (trachea)	Normal—loud, high-pitched, harsh. Expiration ≥ inspiration.
Vesicular (peripheral lung tissue)	Normal—soft, swishing, low-pitched, may sound like a breeze. Inspiration ≥ expiration.
Bronchovesicular (mainstem bronchi)	Normal—soft, blowing. Inspiration = expiration.
Wheezes (can be heard anywhere)	Abnormal—high-pitched, musical, whistling sound. May be heard on inspiration and expiration.
Rhonchi (central airways)	Abnormal—coarse rumbling, low-pitched, snoring sound. May be heard with inspiration and expiration.
Pleural Friction Rub (lateral lung field)	Abnormal—grating or squeaking, may sound like pieces of sandpaper being rubbed together. Heard on inspiration and expiration.
Rales (can be heard anywhere)	Abnormal—soft crackling, bubbling sound.
Stridor (louder in the neck)	Abnormal—high-pitched, crowing sound.

BRONCHITIS, CHRONIC

· ·

CHEST PHYSIOTHERAPY (CPT) PROCEDURE

· ·

Characteristics	Precipitating Factors	Assessment Findings	Nursing Interventions
• Chronic sputum with cough production on a daily basis for 3 months per year • Chronic hypoxia, cor pulmonale • Increased mucus, cilia production • Increased bronchial wall thickness • Reduced responsiveness of respiratory center to hypoxemic stimuli	• Smoking	• Generalized cyanosis • "Blue bloaters" • Right-sided heart failure • Distended neck veins • Crackles • Expiratory wheezes • Dependent edema • Normal weight or overweight	• Lowest FiO_2 possible to prevent CO_2 retention. • Monitor for fluid overload. • Maintain PaO_2 between 55 and 60. • Teach pursed-lip breathing and diaphragmatic breathing. • Teach tripod position. • Administer bronchodilators, corticosteroids, mucolytics, and antibiotics as prescribed. • Instruct client on the proper use of oral and inhaled medications.

. . . .

1. Perform during morning hours, 1 hour prior to meals or 2 to 3 hours after meals.
2. If the client experiences pain, stop immediately.
3. If the client is receiving tube feedings, stop the feedings and aspirate the residual before beginning therapy.
4. Administer bronchodilator medication 15 minutes before (if indicated).
5. Assure there is a layer of material between the hands or percussion device and the client's skin.
6. Position client for postural drainage based on respiratory assessment.
7. Percuss the area for 1 to 2 minutes.
8. Vibrate the same area while the client exhales four to five deep breaths.
9. Monitor client's respiratory status/tolerance for therapy; stop immediately if cyanosis or exhaustion occurs.
10. Have the client maintain the position for 5 to 20 minutes post-therapy.
11. Repeat in all necessary positions until the client no longer expectorates mucus.
12. Properly dispose of sputum.
13. Assist the client with mouth care post-therapy.

. . . .

CONGESTIVE OBSTRUCTIVE PULMONARY DISEASE (COPD)

. . . .

EMPHYSEMA

. . . .

Definition: Refers to a group of lung diseases that block airflow as clients exhale and make it increasingly difficult to breathe. Emphysema and chronic asthmatic bronchitis are the two main conditions that make up this disease. In all cases, damage to the airways eventually interferes with the exchange of oxygen and carbon dioxide in the lungs. This disease is a leading cause of illness and death worldwide. Causes include long-term smoking, and it can be prevented by not smoking or quitting soon after clients start. This damage to the lungs is irreversible; thus, treatment focuses on controlling symptoms and minimizing further lung damage.

Characteristics	Precipitating Factors	Assessment	Nursing Interventions
• Reduced gas-exchange surface area • Increased air trapping • Decreased capillary network • Increased work, increased O_2 consumption	• Cigarette smoking • Environment and/or occupational exposure • Genetic	• "Pink puffers" • Barrel chest • Pursed-lip breathing • Distant, quiet breath sounds • Wheezes • Pulmonary blebs on X-ray • Anorexia with weight loss, thin in appearance • Tripod positioning	• Lowest FiO_2 possible to prevent CO_2 retention. • Monitor for fluid overload. • Maintain PaO_2 between 55 and 60. • Teach pursed-lip breathing and diaphragmatic breathing. • Teach tripod position. • Administer bronchodilators, corticosteroids, mucolytics, and antibiotics as prescribed. • Instruct client on the proper use of oral and inhaled medications.

HEMOTHORAX

. . . .

INCENTIVE SPIROMETRY, CLIENT INSTRUCTIONS FOR

. . . .

LEGIONNAIRES' DISEASE

Definition: Presence of blood in the pleural cavity related to trauma or a ruptured aortic aneurysm.

· ·

1. Instruct the client to take a sitting upright position.
2. Instruct the client to place his or her mouth tightly around the mouth-piece of the device.
3. Instruct the client to inhale slowly to raise and maintain the flow rate indicator between the 600 to 900 markings.
4. Instruct the client to hold his or her breath for 5 seconds and then exhale through pursed lips.
5. Instruct the client to repeat the process 10 times every hour.

· ·

Definition: A severe form of pneumonia; lung inflammation usually caused by infection.

Causes: *Legionella pneumophila* and inhaling bacteria. Older adults, smokers, and clients with weakened immune systems are particularly susceptible. Sources of the organism include contaminated cooling water and warm stagnant water supplies, including water vaporizers, water sonicators, showers, and whirlpool spas.

Assessment Findings: Influenza-like symptoms with chills, high fever, muscle aches, and headache that may progress to pleurisy, dry cough, and occasionally diarrhea.

Treatment/Nursing Interventions: Treatment is supportive. Antibiotic therapy may be initiated.

Special Considerations: The risk for infection is increased by the presence of other conditions. Left untreated, Legionnaires' disease can be fatal.

LUNG CANCER

. . . .

MECHANICAL VENTILATION, CONTROLS AND SETTINGS, I

. . . .

Definition: Malignant tumor of the bronchi and peripheral lung tissue. The lungs are a common target for metastasis from other organs. There are two main types of lung cancer based on histological cell type, small cell lung cancer (SCLC) and non–small cell lung cancer (NSCLC).

Causes: Cigarette smoking, occupational exposure to and/or inhalation of carcinogens.

Assessment Findings: Can be nonspecific; symptoms appear late in the disease. Dyspnea, pain on swallowing, chronic cough, hoarseness, hemoptysis, chest pain, anorexia and weight loss, weakness, recurring fever.

Treatment/Nursing Interventions: Radiation, chemotherapy, lobectomy, pneumonectomy, lung conserving resection. Treatment can include all three therapies: radiation, chemotherapy, and surgery.

Controls and Settings	Description
Tidal Volume	The volume of air that the client receives with each breath.
Rate	The number of breaths delivered by the ventilator per minute.
Sighs	The volume of air that is 1.5 to 2 times the set tidal volume, delivered 6 to 10 times per hour; may be initiated to prevent atelectasis.
Fraction of Inspired Oxygen (FiO$_2$)	The oxygen concentration delivered to the client; determined by the client's medical status and arterial blood gas (ABG) results.

MECHANICAL VENTILATION, CONTROLS AND SETTINGS, II

Controls and Settings	Description
Peak Airway Inspiratory Pressure	The pressure required by the ventilator to deliver a set tidal volume at a given compliance. Monitoring peak airway inspiratory pressure reflects changes in compliance of the lungs and resistance in the ventilator or the client.
Continuous Positive Airway Pressure	The application of positive airway pressure throughout the entire respiratory cycle for spontaneously breathing clients. Acts to keep the alveoli open during inspiration and prevents alveolar collapse; used primarily as a weaning modality. No ventilator breaths are delivered, but the ventilator delivers oxygen and provides monitor and an alarm system; the respiratory pattern is determined by the client's efforts.
Positive End-Expiratory Pressure (PEEP)	Positive pressure is exerted during the expiratory phase of ventilation, which improves oxygenation by enhancing gas exchange and preventing atelectasis. When a client is placed on PEEP, this indicates a severe gas-exchange disturbance. Higher amounts of PEEP ≥15 increase the chance for the client to experience barotraumas and/or a pneumothorax.
Pressure Support	The oxygen concentration delivered to the client; determined by the client's medical status and arterial blood gas (ABG) results.

MECHANICAL VENTILATION, MODES OF

. . . .

PNEUMONIA

. . . .

Controlled	Least-used mode. The client receives a set tidal volume at a set rate; used in clients who cannot initiate respiratory effort; if the client attempts to initiate a breath, the ventilator blocks the effort.
Assist-Control (AC)	Most commonly used mode. Tidal volume and ventilatory rate are preset on the ventilator. Ventilator takes over the work of breathing for the client, is programmed to respond to the client's inspiratory effort if the client does initiate a breath, and delivers the preset tidal volume when the client initiates a breath while allowing the client to control the rate of breathing. If the client's spontaneous ventilatory rate increases, the ventilator continues to deliver a preset tidal volume with each breath, which may cause hyperventilation and respiratory alkalosis.
Synchronized Intermittent Mandatory Ventilation (SIMV)	Similar to AC in that the tidal volume and ventilatory rate are preset on the ventilator. SIMV permits the client to breathe spontaneously at his or her own rate and tidal volume between the ventilator breaths. Can be utilized as the primary mode or as a weaning mode. When used as a weaning mode, the number of SIMV breaths is decreased gradually, and the client gradually resumes spontaneous breathing.

· ·

Definition: An acute inflammatory process caused by a microbial agent; it involves the lung parenchyma, including the small airways and alveoli. The edema associated with inflammation stiffens the lung, decreases lung capacity, and causes hypoxia. It can be community-acquired or hospital-acquired.

Causes: Predisposing conditions: chronic upper respiratory infections, smoking, aspiration of foreign or gastric content. Viral causes: influenza, parainfluenza; Bacterial causes: *Streptococcus pneumonias*, *Mycoplasma pneumonia*, *Staphylococcus aureus*.

Assessment Findings: Fever, chills, tachycardia, dyspnea, productive cough (thick, blood-streaked, yellow, purulent sputum), chest pains, respiratory distress, ronchi, and wheezing.

Treatment/Nursing Interventions: Position client in high Fowler's position, respiratory precautions as indicated; cool mist O_2; postural drainage; administer bronchodilators, antipyretics, antibiotics, bronchodilators, cough suppressants, mucolytic agents, and expectorants as prescribed; encourage coughing and deep-breathing exercises and the use of incentive spirometer; and provide chest physical therapy.

Special Considerations: Teach the client the importance of proper hand washing, disposing of respiratory secretions properly, and receiving vaccinations such as the flu and pneumonia immunizations.

· ·

PNEUMOTHORAX

PART II

· ·

PULMONARY EMBOLISM (PE)

· ·

Definition: Presence of air within the pleural cavity; occurs spontaneously or as a result of trauma. Pressure builds up in the pleural space, lung on the affected side collapses, and the heart and mediastinum shift toward the unaffected lung. There are three types: open, spontaneous, and tension. *Open* occurs when an opening through the chest wall allows the entrance of positive atmospheric air pressure into the pleural space. *Spontaneous* occurs with the rupture of a pulmonary bleb. *Tension* occurs from blunt trauma to the chest wall or mechanical ventilation with positive end-expiratory pressure (PEEP) when a buildup of positive pressure occurs in the pleural space.

. . . .

Definition: Movement of a thrombus from its original site of origin to the lungs.
Causes: Prolonged immobility, advanced age, surgery (especially joint replacements of the hip and knee), heart disease, cancer, pregnancy, smoking, obesity, supplemental estrogen.
Assessment Findings: *Mild:* Mimic those of pleurisy or bronchial pneumonia, dyspnea, pleuritic pain, tachycardia, elevated temperature, cough with hemoptysis. *Severe:* Chest pain, severe dyspnea leading to air hunger, shallow rapid respirations, sharp substernal chest pain, vertigo leading to syncope, hypovolemia, cardiac dysrhythmias, weakness, severe anxiety, and hypotension.
Treatment/Nursing Interventions: Maintain patent airway; place client in high Fowler's position; apply oxygen as ordered (assist with intubation as indicated); monitor pulse oximetry, arterial blood gases, and breath sounds; encourage client to cough and deep breathe. Vital signs every 2 to 4 hours; turn and reposition client as ordered; administer anticoagulants (i.e., heparin IV), diuretics, and narcotic as prescribed. For acute right-ventricular failure or refractory hypoxia, administer thrombolytics (i.e., t-PA, streptokinanse); surgical intervention (femoral vein ligation, pulmonary embolectomy, vein filter) is indicated when client is unresponsive to heparin therapy.
Special Considerations: Prevention measures: ambulate client as soon as possible after surgery, complete range of motion exercises, and apply compression stockings.

. . . .

TUBERCULOSIS (TB)

. . . .

TUBERCULOSIS, CLIENT EDUCATION FOR

. . . .

Definition: An inflammatory, highly communicable disease that most commonly attacks the lungs, although it can occur in other parts of the body (brain, kidney, liver, joints, intestines, and peritoneum).

Causes: *Mycobacterium tuberculosis*, a gram-positive, acid-fast bacillus.

Assessment Findings: Up to 20% of clients may be asymptomatic. Subjective data includes loss of appetite, weight loss; weakness, loss of energy; pain: knifelike in the chest; client may be asymptomatic, but disease is found through screening measure. Objective data: night sweats; low-grade, late afternoon fever; tachycardia; productive cough with hemoptysis; increased depth of respirations; asymmetrical lung expansion; increased tactile fremitus; and crackles following short cough.

Treatment/Nursing Interventions: Administer commonly used medications as directed (isoniazid/INH, rifampin/rifadin), avoid direct contact with sputum, promote nutrition, increase client self-esteem, promote health teaching, and ensure respiratory isolation.

Special Considerations: Respiratory isolation for infectious diseases is critical. Clients must be assessed for their ability to comply with prescribed therapy. Diagnosis is based on a variety of factors, including chest assessment, chest x-ray, QuantiFERON-TB Gold test, sputum cultures, and the Mantoux skin test.

. . . .

1. Speak to client and family about the contagious aspect of the infection and provide the client/family with information about TB.
2. Relay to client/family to follow the medication regimen exactly as prescribed.
3. Discuss with client/family the side effects related to the medication regimen, and ways of minimizing them to obtain/assure compliance.
4. Offer the client/family reassurance that after 2 to 3 weeks of medication therapy, they will likely not be able to affect anyone.
5. Reassure the client/family that resuming activities gradually is acceptable.
6. Instruct client/family about the importance for adequate nutrition in an effort to promote healing.
7. Inform the client and family that respiratory isolation is not necessary because family members have already been exposed.
8. Direct client to cover mouth and nose when coughing and sneezing and to dispose of tissues in a plastic bag.
9. Instruct client that once medication regimen is begun, a sputum culture is needed every 2 to 4 weeks.
10. Inform the client that once the results of three sputum cultures are negative, he or she is no longer considered infectious and can resume working.

. . . .

NCLEX-RN Flash Review

TUBERCULOSIS, RISK FACTORS/CAUSES OF

. . . .

Individuals who have been exposed to tubercle bacillus
Children ≤5 years old
Men ≥65 years old
Women between the ages of 22 and 44 and ≥65 years of age
Individuals who abuse alcohol or use intravenous drugs
Individuals in institutions (e.g., prisons, long-term facilities, and mental health facilities)
Homeless individuals, or those from minority, refugee, or lower socioeconomic groups
Individuals with malnutrition, immune dysfunction, human immunodeficiency virus or other infection, or who are immunosuppressed as a result of medication therapy

Part III

OBSTETRICS

BALLOTTEMENT

· ·

BISHOP SCORE

· ·

BRAXTON HICKS CONTRACTIONS

Definition: Passive movement of the fetus that occurs when the lower segment of the uterine wall is tapped during a bimanual exam. The fetus rises and can be felt as it touches the abdominal wall. Ballottement is a probable sign of pregnancy.

· ·

	0	1	2	3
Cervical Dilation (cm)	0	1–2	3–4	>5
Cervical Effacement (%)	0–30	40–50	60–70	>80
Cervical Consistency	Firm	Medium	Soft	—
Cervical Position	Posterior	Midposition	Anterior	—
Presenting Part Station	–3	–2	–1	+1 to +2

A total score of 8 or greater indicates that the cervix is ready for induction of labor.

· ·

Definition: Uterine contractions that are mild, irregular, and typically not felt in the back. They begin early in the pregnancy and increase in frequency after 28 weeks. Unlike contractions of true labor, Braxton Hicks contractions *do not* cause cervical effacement or dilation, and they can be diminished by eating, changing positions, or ambulating.

CHADWICK'S SIGN

....

GOODELL'S SIGN

....

GTPAL

Definition: A bluish discoloration of the vagina, cervix, and vulva that can be observed at approximately 6 to 8 weeks' gestation. It is considered a probable sign of pregnancy.

· ·

Definition: A softening of the cervix that can be felt at approximately 6 to 8 weeks' gestation. It is considered to be a probable sign of pregnancy.

· ·

	Term	Definition
G	Gravida	Number of times that a woman has been pregnant, including current pregnancy
T	Term	Number of pregnancies carried to term (≤38 weeks)
P	Para	Number of infants delivered at or above the age of viability (approximately 20 to 24 weeks)
A	Abortion	Number of times a pregnancy was ended by abortion, either spontaneous or induced
L	Living	Number of children currently alive

HEGAR'S SIGN

· ·

MORNING SICKNESS/HYPEREMESIS GRAVIDARUM

· ·

NAEGELE'S RULE

Definition: Softening of the lower segment of the uterine consistency. It is considered to be a probable sign of pregnancy.

• •

	Morning Sickness	Hyperemesis Gravidarum
Signs and Symptoms	Transient nausea occurring anytime during day. Usually diminishes after first month but may be present throughout the pregnancy.	Severe nausea and vomiting. Dehydration. Decreased weight. Oliguria. Electrolyte imbalance.
Treatment	Dry crackers 15 minutes before getting out of bed. Small frequent meals. Water between meals, not with meals. Avoid smells/foods that cause nausea.	Cessation of nausea and vomiting. IV fluids. Electrolyte replacement. Eating guidelines for morning sickness.

• •

Definition: Utilized to determine the estimated due date (EDD) by employing the following steps:

- Determine the first day of the woman's last menstrual period (LMP).
- Add 1 year.
- Subtract 3 months.
- Add 7 days to that date.

Example: LMP first day plus 1 year   March 8
             Subtract three months   December 8
             Add seven days   December 15
             EDD   December 15

PART III

NUTRITION

....

PRENATAL VISITS

....

PSYCHOLOGICAL TASKS

Calories	Increase by 300 calories per day
Protein/Meat	2–3 3-ounce servings/day
Breads/Grains	6–11 servings/day
Fruits	2–4 servings/day
Vegetables	4+ servings/day
Dairy	4 servings/day
Folic Acid	600–800 mcg/day
Vitamin C	70–85 mg/day
Foods to Avoid	Raw or undercooked eggs and meats Raw fish Swordfish, king mackerel, tilefish, shark Soft cheeses Alcohol Street drugs Tobacco
Foods to Limit	Caffeine to 300 mg/day

. . . .

Gestational Week(s)	Frequency
4 through 32	Monthly
32–36	Every other week
36 until Labor/Delivery	Weekly
Assessments	Urine analysis for albumen, glucose, protein Weight Fundal height (after 12 to 13 weeks) Fetal heart rate (after 10 to 12 weeks) Signs and/or symptoms of discomforts of pregnancy Signs and/or symptoms of complications Anticipatory guidance

. . . .

First Trimester	• Resolve any ambivalence about pregnancy. • Maternal acceptance of physical changes. • Paternal acceptance of impending fatherhood.
Second Trimester	• Development of prenatal attachment. • Mother and father image development.
Third Trimester	• Prepare for birth experience. • Prepare for parenting. • Accept body image.

QUICKENING

· ·

RH INCOMPATIBILITY

PART III

· ·

SIGNS OF PREGNANCY

Definition: Quickening refers to the first fetal movements that are felt by the mother. Pregnant women often describe the sensation as a "fluttering" or "bubbling." Quickening occurs between the 16th and 26th weeks of pregnancy, but most frequently is experienced between the 18th and 22nd week. Quickening is considered to be a presumptive sign of pregnancy.

• •

Definition: Also known as isoimmunization, Rh incompatibility occurs when the pregnant woman is Rh-negative and her fetus is Rh-positive. Usually the Rh-negative woman carries her first Rh-positive child without incident, unless she is exposed to the fetal blood.
Causes: Rh-positive blood cells from the fetus enter the maternal blood circulation, causing maternal sensitization through the formation of antigens. The antigens then cross the placenta and enter the fetal blood stream, causing hemolysis, hypoxia, and fetal death.
Assessment Findings: Anti-D antibody titer of 1.16 or greater.
Treatment: The goal of treatment is to prevent Rh isoimmunization from occurring. RhoGAM is usually given at 28 weeks' gestation and after exposure to fetal blood. It is also given within 72 hours of delivery.
Special Consideration: The woman should also be given a card to carry identifying her as Rh-negative.

• •

Type	Signs/Symptoms
Presumptive Signs	Breast tenderness, tingling, enlargement Morning sickness Missed period (amenorrhea) Frequent urination Fatigue Quickening Striae gravidarum (stretch marks)
Probable Signs	Goodell's sign Hegar's sign Chadwick's sign Ballottement Braxton Hicks contractions
Positive Signs	Fetal heart beat Sonographic evidence of fetus Palpation of fetal movement through abdomen

SYSTEM, CARDIOVASCULAR

. . . .

SYSTEM, GASTROINTESTINAL

. . . .

SYSTEM, GENITOURINARY

PART III

Heart Rate	• Increases 10–15 beats/min. in second trimester • Increases 15–20 beats/min. in third trimester
Ausculatory	• Split S1 may be noticed. • S3 may be heard after 20 weeks' gestation.
Blood Pressure	• Considered within normal limits if less than 140/90.
Blood Volume	• Increases by approximately 40%.
Cardiac Output	• Increases by 50% due to increased tissue demand and increased stroke volume. • Side-lying position increases cardiac output. • Lying on back decreases cardiac output.
Coagulation	• Coagulation factor I increases by 50% to prevent maternal hemorrhage during childbirth but also puts woman at risk for deep vein thrombosis (DVT).

• •

Gums	• Increased vascularity may cause gums to become edematous and bleed easily.
Stomach	• Mobility decreases, causing an increase in emptying time. • As uterine enlarges, it displaces the stomach and further slows emptying time. • Acidity decreases. • Delayed emptying time may lead to heartburn.
Intestines	• Mobility decreases. • Uterine enlargement displaces intestines, slowing peristalsis. • May lead to heartburn, constipation, flatulence, hemorrhoids.
Gallbladder	• Emptying time increases. • Increased tendency for gallstones.

• •

Bladder	• Urinary frequency in the first and last trimesters.
Kidneys	• Increased glomerular filtration leads to increased filtration of glucose, which sometimes is excreted into urine. Finding more than a trace of glucose in the urine is considered abnormal.
Uterus	Increases in size.
Cervix	• Softens. • Vascularity increases, causing the cervix to take on a bluish hue (Chadwick's sign). • Pregnant women may notice bleeding after sexual activity.
Vagina	• Develops bluish hue. • Pregnant women are prone to yeast infections due to increased acidity of vaginal secretions.

SYSTEM, INTEGUMENTARY

· ·

SYSTEM, MUSCULOSKELETAL

· ·

SYSTEM, RESPIRATORY

Straie Gravidarum	• Stretch marks. • Appear as pink or red streaks.
Linea Nigra	• Dark line that forms from the umbilicus to the mons pubis.
Melasma	• Darkened areas that form on the cheeks and nose after the 16th week. • Also known as the "Mask of Pregnancy."
Palmar Erythema	• Pinkish areas over the palmar surface of the hands.
Epulides	• Raised, red, painful areas on the gums.
Nevi	• Bright red angiomas.

Rectal Abdominal Diastasis	Separation of rectus abdominal muscle can occur due to stretching of abdominal wall to accommodate increasing size of uterus.
Pelvic, Sacroiliac, Sacrococcygeal Joints	Relaxation of the joints causes changes in posture and gait; relaxation of the pelvis may lead to increased pain in nul-lipara women.
Wrist	Carpal tunnel syndrome may occur.

Respiratory Rate	May increase by two breaths per minute above baseline during third trimester. Shortness of breath (SOB) often common due to decreased ability of diaphragm to expand because of increasing size of uterus.
Epitaxis	May occur due to increased vascularization of upper respiratory tract.

WEIGHT GAIN

· ·

WEIGHT GAIN DISTRIBUTION

· ·

Recommended weight gains:

Normal Weight Prepregnancy	25 to 32 pounds
Underweight Prepregnancy	27 to 39 pounds
Overweight Prepregnancy*	15 to 25 pounds

*Weight loss during pregnancy is discouraged.

· ·

Weight in Pounds	
2	Amniotic fluid
4–5	Blood volume
1–4	Breasts
3–5	Extracellular fluid
7–8	Fetus (average weight)
2–2.5	Placenta
2	Uterus

Remainder of weight gain is deposited in maternal fat stores.

· ·

AMNIOTIC FLUID CHARACTERISTICS

. . . .

CARDINAL MOVEMENTS OF LABOR

. . . .

CERVICAL DILATION

Amount at Term	Normal: Oliohydramnios: Polyhydramnios:	Between 500 BS 1,000 mL Less than 500 mL Greater than 2,000 mL
Character	Normal: Infection:	Thin Thick
Odor	Normal: Infection:	Odorless Odor present
Color	Normal: Fetal distress: Abruptio placenta: Infection:	Clear; white flecks may be present Green or meconium stained Port-wine Yellow

. . . .

Descent	Downward movement of the fetus.
Flexion	Fetal head bends to chest to present the smallest diameter.
Internal Rotation	Head enters pelvis, then rotates 90 degrees so that the back of the neck can proceed under symphysis.
Extension	Head passes through pelvis through symphysis pubis. Upward resistance from pelvic floor causes head to extend, allowing occiput, brow, face, and chin to emerge.
External Rotation	Turning of shoulders so that they are in anteroposterior diameter of pelvis; the shoulders are then delivered.
Expulsion	Birth of entire body.

. . . .

Definition: Refers to the opening of the cervix from 0 to 10 cm to accommodate delivery of the fetus. Cervix dilation occurs during the first phase of labor.

CERVICAL EFFACEMENT

. . . .

CESAREAN DELIVERY

. . . .

PAIN RELIEF: NONPHARMACOLOGICAL

Definition: Refers to the thinning of the cervix during the labor process. Effacement progressively shortens the cervix until there is no length and it is paper thin. Occurs during the first phase of labor.

. . . .

Definition: Surgical birth of the fetus; may be planned or unplanned.
Causes: Placenta previa; premature separation of membranes (PROM); transverse or breech presentation; cephalopelvic disproportion; active genital herpes; previous cesarean birth; fetal distress; preeclampsia/eclampsia; inadequate progression of labor.
Assessment Findings: Ultrasonography reveals malposition of fetus, cephalopelvic disproportion, fetal distress.
Nursing Interventions: *Pre-op:* Educate and provide support to parents; if planned C-section, complete preoperative teaching; begin IV infusion, type and cross match as ordered. *Post-op:* Fundal checks; check perineal pad and abdominal dressing; ensure mother/infant bonding; monitor vital signs, including pain level; encourage cough and deep breathing, as well as early ambulation.
Special Consideration: Allow mother to see, touch, and hold infant as soon after delivery as possible to promote bonding.

. . . .

Relaxation Techniques	Positioning. Focusing and imagery. Therapeutic touch. Music therapy. Support of birthing partner. Most effective in the early phases of labor.
Breathing Techniques/ Lamaze Method	Each type of breathing starts and ends with deep, cleansing breaths; includes slow, deep breaths in and out, pant-blow pattern "he-he-he-hoo," and/or continuous panting.

PAIN RELIEF: PHARMACOLOGICAL

·····

PASSAGEWAY

·····

PASSENGER

Opioids	Demoral, stadol, nubain, sublimaze; may relax cervix; may depress central nervous system of fetus.
Meperidine	Given IM, IV, or intrathecally; sedative and antispasmodic; given when woman is more than 3 hours from birth to prevent fetal respiratory depression.
Regional Nerve Block	Can lower woman's BP; may slow labor if given before 5 cm dilation; may decrease bearing-down reflex and ability to push.
Epidural	Used in first and second stages; usually preserves bearing-down reflex; if contractions become less frequent, intense, or shorter in duration, notify MD immediately; position woman in modified Sims to receive the epidural.
Pudendal	Short duration; used for actual birth and perineal repair; does not depress neonate but may inhibit bearing-down reflex.

· ·

Definition: One of the four Ps or major factors that interact for a safe delivery, it refers to the birth canal. The subpubic angle of the pelvis must be wide enough to allow the presenting part of the fetus to pass under it. Pelvic shapes include:

Gynecoid:	Round	Conducive to vaginal birth
Platypelloid:	Flat	Conducive to vaginal birth
Android:	Heart	Not conducive to vaginal birth
Anthropoid:	Oval	Not conducive to vaginal birth

· ·

One of the four Ps or major factors that interact for a safe delivery, it refers to:

Presentation	First fetal part entering into pelvic inlet. *Cephalic:* Head first; most common. *Breech:* May need cesarean section: Complete: Feet and legs flexed; buttocks and feet present. Frank: Feet up on shoulders; buttocks present. Footling: One or both feet present.
Fetal Lie	Relationship of fetal spine to maternal spine: *Transverse:* Shoulder presents. *Longitudinal:* Vertex or breech presentation.
Attitude	Relationship of fetal parts to one another. Example: Fetal head flexed to chest.
Position	Relationship of presenting part to quadrants within maternal pelvis. Example: Anterior occipital on maternal left side (LOA).

POWERS OF LABOR

. . . .

PSYCHE

. . . .

SIGNS OF IMPENDING LABOR

PART
III

Definition: One of the four Ps or major factors that interact to allow a safe delivery, it refers to the strength and effectiveness of uterine contractions.

· ·

Definition: One of the four Ps or major factors that interact for a safe delivery, it refers to the woman's emotional state during labor. The emotional response of a woman impacts her physiological and psychological functioning during labor and may impede or facilitate the labor process.

· ·

Lightening	Engagement of the fetal head in the pelvis; takes place two weeks before labor in primiparas but often not until labor begins in multiparas; may cause increased pressure on the bladder, resulting in urinary frequency.
Nesting	Urge to clean the house, prepare the nursery, or do other things to prepare the "nest" for the arrival of the baby.
Braxton Hicks	Increase in strength and frequency.
Decreased Weight	Hormonal changes decrease water retention.
Bloody Show	Passage of blood-tinged mucous from the vagina; labor may begin in 24 to 48 hours.
Cervical Changes	Cervix is shorter, softer, and may be dilated 1 to 2 cm.
Rupture of Membranes	May be a gush or a trickle; mother should be advised to come to hospital, as labor may begin within 24 hours.

STAGE OF LABOR, FIRST

. . . .

STAGE OF LABOR, SECOND

. . . .

STAGE OF LABOR, THIRD

First Stage of Labor	Begins with onset of true labor and ends when cervix is completely effaced and dilated to 10 cm.
Latent Phase	Contractions are regular with a frequency of 5–15 minutes, duration of 10–30 seconds, and mild intensity; station –2 to –1.
Active Phase	Cervix dilates from 3 or 4 cm to 8 cm. Fetus descends through birth canal to 0 or +1 station. Contractions 3–5 minutes apart with duration of 30–45 seconds, moderate intensity.
Transition Phase	Cervix dilates from 8 to 10 cm. Contractions occur every 1.5 to 2 minutes, last 60–90 seconds, and have a strong intensity. Station +1 to +2.
Nursing Interventions	Assess vital signs, contractions, fetal heart rate, bladder distension, cervical changes; keep NPO (nothing by mouth); reinforce breathing/relaxation techniques; care for symptoms; administer pain medications as ordered; provide support.

• •

Definition: From cervical dilation of 10 cm to delivered infant.
Assessment Findings: Contractions every 2 to 3 minutes lasting 60 to 90 seconds; maternal urge to push; visibility of presenting part; bulging perineum; increased bloody show.
Nursing Interventions: Monitor maternal vital signs and fetal heart rate; pad stirrups, raise both legs simultaneously into stirrups; cleanse vulva and perineum as needed; provide oxygen if decreased fetal heart rate; encourage mother to take a deep breath before pushing and to push as long as possible with each contraction; involve father: where to stand, what is occurring.
Special Consideration: Mother may need to be catheterized if distended bladder prevents fetal descent.

• •

Definition: Delivery of infant to delivery of placenta.
Assessment Findings: Signs of placental separation: Umbilical cord lengthens; uterus rises upward in abdomen and changes shape; sudden trickle of blood.
Nursing Interventions: Position infant with mother to encourage eye-to-eye contact and bonding; provide support to parents; splint or support abdomen as mother expels placenta; inspect placenta to ensure that it is intact. Assess fundus: should be midline and just below umbilicus.
Special Considerations: Maternal trembling common: no clinical significance. Umbilical cord should have two arteries and one vein.

STAGE OF LABOR, FOURTH

. . . .

STATION

. . . .

TIMING CONTRACTIONS

Definition: Expulsion of placenta 1 to 4 hours after delivery of fetus.
Assessment Findings: Firm fundus; BP returns to predelivery level; pulse slightly lower than during delivery.
Nursing Interventions: Assess maternal vital signs; assess amount and character of vaginal blood flow; assess fundus for location, firmness. Assist woman to stand for first of several times and assist with ambulation. Provide comfort and support.
Special Considerations: Lowered blood pressure and rising pulse may be indicative of increased blood loss.

· ·

Denotes the relationship between the presenting fetal part and the ischial spine of the maternal pelvis. The following table identifies and defines common terms related to station:

0 Station	Presenting part is at level of the spines.
–1, –2, –3 Station	Level of presenting part is above spines in cm.
+1, +2, +3 Station	Level of presenting part is below spines in cm.
High Station	Presenting part is not engaged.
Floating	Presenting part is able to move freely within pelvis.
Dipping	Entering into pelvis.
Engaged	Presenting part passed through pelvic inlet.
Fixed	No longer movable; engaged.

· ·

Definition: To determine the *frequency* of contractions, time it from the beginning of one contraction to the beginning of the next. To determine the *duration* of a contraction, time it from the beginning of the contraction to the end of the contraction.

TRUE VERSUS FALSE LABOR

	True Labor	False Labor
Contractions	• Regular. • Increase in intensity with ambulation. • Increase in duration and frequency. • From back spreading to abdomen.	• Irregular. • Decreases in intensity with ambulation. • No changes in duration and frequency. • Localized in abdomen.
Cervix	• Progressively dilates and effaces.	• No cervical changes.
Bloody Show	• Present.	• Not present.

ASSESSMENT/NURSING INTERVENTIONS IN POSTPARTUM PERIOD

. . . .

BONDING PHASES (RUBIN'S)

. . . .

FUNDAL ASSESSMENT

Assessment	• Vital signs, intake and outputs (I&O), return of bowel functioning. • Fundus, lochia, perineum, episiostomy, hemorrhoids. • Breasts for engorgement, cracked or inverted nipples. • Legs for DVTs. • Bonding with infant.
Nursing Interventions	• Administer RhoGAM if needed (Rh-neg mom, Rh-pos infant). • Perform/teach perineal care. • Encourage ambulation. • Discuss return to sexual activity and contraception if client desires. • Teach infant care, including breast-/bottle-feeding, bathing infant, care of cord, and circumcision site (if needed). • Promote parental-infant bonding.

Phase	Description	Nursing Interventions
Taking-In	Mother focused on her needs and on her delivery experience.	Encourage verbalization.
Taking-Hold	Mother feels more in control and ready to begin caring for infant.	Teach infant care.
Letting-Go	Mother may feel guilty/resentful about the amount of work involved in caring for infant; may feel conflict over role of mother and wife; may develop postpartum blues or postpartum depression.	Encourage verbalization of feelings. Offer positive reinforcement. Assess for s/s depression and make appropriate referrals as needed.

The fundus is assessed for consistency and location. Findings include:

Immediately postdelivery	Firm; 1–2 cm below umbilicus
12 hours postpartum	Firm; 1 cm above umbilicus
24 hours postpartum	Firm; 1 cm below umbilicus
48 hours postpartum	Firm; 2 cm below umbilicus
9 days postpartum	No longer palpable

Special Consideration: The fundus moves below the umbilicus at a rate of 1 cm per day. If the fundus is soft or boggy, it should be gently massaged with fingertips.

LOCHIA

Definition: Refers to the vaginal drainage during the postpartum period. It should be without clots and foul odor. During the first 1 to 3 days postpartum, it should be red in color (*lochia rubra*). From day 3 through 7 it should be pink (*lochia serosa*). From day 7 to 10 it should be creamy white (*lochia alba*).

• •

NCLEX-RN Flash Review

ABRUPTIO PLACENTA

. . . .

ANEMIA

. . . .

DISSEMINATED INTRAVASCULAR COAGULATION (DIC)

PART
III

Definition: Separation of placenta from implantation site prior to birth of fetus.
Causes: Trauma, preeclampsia, eclampsia, illicit drugs, chronic vascular renal disease.
Assessment Findings: Abdominal pain with dark red vaginal bleeding.
Nursing Interventions: Keep patient on bed rest; monitor vital signs, PT and PTT, central venous pressure, and urinary output; monitor fetus; obtain order for type, and cross match blood for possible transfusion; administer IV as per order; assess for disseminated intravascular coagulation (DIC).
Special Considerations: Three types of separation may occur: *complete* (complete separation); *partial* (only a portion is separated); or *central* (central portion is separated, causing blood to pool behind placenta and uterine wall, concealing the bleeding).

Definition: Deficient hemoglobin synthesis, impairing transport of oxygen.
Causes: Inadequate maternal iron stores and/or inadequate oral iron intake.
Assessment Findings: Fatigue, headaches, pallor, tachycardia, shortness of breath, hemoglobin <10 g/dL and hematocrit <30%; dry skin at corners of the mouth; tongue that is sore and red.
Nursing Interventions: Monitor hemoglobin and hematocrit; instruct client to take iron supplement as ordered and with vitamin C to increase absorption but instruct client to avoid taking iron supplement with tea; instruct client to eat foods high in iron, folic acid, and protein.
Special Consideration: Compliance with taking prescription prenatal vitamins, which can prevent anemia.

Definition: Maternal condition in which simultaneous activation of fibrinolytic and thrombin systems are activated, causing clots in microcirculation and depletion of clotting factors.
Causes: Abruption placenta, preeclampsia, eclampsia, amniotic fluid embolism, fetal death, liver disease, sepsis.
Assessment Findings: Excessive ecchymosis; uncontrolled bleeding; hematuria; hematemesis; vaginal bleeding; shock; decreased fibrinogen level, platelet count, and hematocrit with increased PT, PTT.
Nursing Interventions: Assess/monitor vital signs, urinary output, bleeding, and s/s shock; initiate oxygen therapy; administer blood component therapy as ordered; assist in carrying out MD orders for treatment of underlying cause.
Special Considerations: Complications of DIC include renal failure: report urine output < than 30 mL/hour to physician.

ECLAMPSIA

....

ECTOPIC PREGNANCY

....

GESTATIONAL DIABETES

Definition: A severe form of pregnancy-induced hypertension.
Cause: Risk factors include nullipara women.
Assessment Findings: Severe preeclampsia plus onset of seizure activity or convulsions.
Nursing Interventions: Position patient in left-side lying position; maintain patent airway; administer oxygen; after seizure, insert oral airway and suction as needed; administer magnesium sulfate and other medications per order; prepare for delivery via cesarean section (if needed).
Special Consideration: Seizure activity typically begins with uncontrolled twitching of the mouth.

. . . .

Definition: Implantation of the embryo anywhere NOT inside the uterus; most common location is fallopian tube.
Causes: Fertilized ovum's passage through fallopian tubes is slowed or prevented due to fallopian tube obstruction and/or malformation; abdominal adhesions; tubal spasms; previous tubal surgery; diverticuli, or transmigration of ovum to opposite tube.
Assessment Findings: Amenorrhea with slight vaginal bleeding and unilateral pelvic pain; may have referred right shoulder pain, lightheadedness.
Nursing Interventions: Assess vital signs, vaginal bleeding; assess for s/s hypovolemic shock; administer blood transfusions as ordered; prepare patient for laproscopic surgery or administration of methotrexate to stop cell reproduction; encourage verbalization and provide support.
Special Consideration: If patient is Rh-negative, may need RhoGAM after treatment or surgery.

. . . .

Definition: Inability to produce/metabolize enough insulin during pregnancy.
Causes: Predisposing factors include maternal age >35 years; obesity; multiple gestation; family history of diabetes.
Assessment Findings: Increased hunger, thirst, urination, yeast infections, urinary tract infections; weight loss; fetus large for gestational age; glycosuria.
Nursing Interventions: Monitor maternal weight, fetal growth; teach/monitor self glucose testing, diet and exercise regime, s/s management of hypo- and hyperglycemic episodes; assess for s/s yeast infection and/or urinary tract infection; monitor for hypoglycemic reaction postdelivery as insulin requirements sharply decline in the first 24 hours after delivery.
Special Consideration: All women are screened for gestational diabetes during 24 to 28 weeks' gestation via oral glucose challenge testing.

GESTATIONAL HYPERTENSION

. . . .

HELLP SYNDROME

. . . .

HYDATIDIFORM MOLE

Definition: A mild type of pregnancy-induced hypertension occurring after 20 weeks of gestation.
Causes: Risk factors include primigravida, age <19 and >40; diabetes mellitus, Rh incompatibility.
Assessment Findings: BP >140/90 on two separate readings at least 6 hours apart but WITHOUT proteinuria.
Nursing Interventions: Monitor BP, renal function studies, fetal heart tones, and fetal growth. Teach patient monitoring of self BP, medication regime, frequent rest periods in the left lateral lying position.
Special Consideration: Lack of proteinuria is what distinguishes gestational hypertension from preeclampsia

• •

Definition: Gestational hypertension that involves hemolysis, elevated liver enzymes, and low platelets.
Causes: Women with severe preeclampsia and eclampsia are at higher risk.
Assessment Findings: RUQ, epigastric, or lower chest pain; nausea and vomiting; severe edema; s/s preeclampsia/eclampsia; blood smear reveals hemolysis of red blood cells; thrombocytopenia; elevated liver enzymes.
Nursing Interventions: Assess maternal vital signs and fetal heart rate; assess for complications, including hemorrhage, renal failure, hypoglycemia; initiate bleeding precautions and administer blood products as ordered; administer magnesium sulfate as ordered; prepare woman for delivery.
Special Consideration: Do NOT palpate abdomen.

• •

Definition: Disease in which tropoblasts develop abnormally and manifest as a grapelike cluster of cells. Also known as tropoblastic disease and molar pregnancy.
Causes: Not known.
Assessment Findings: Vaginal bleeding, fundal height greater than for gestational age; no fetal heart rate; ultrasound reveals "snowstorm" pattern versus fetus.
Nursing Interventions: Prepare woman for evacuation of hydatidiform mole by vacuum aspiration; administer oxytocin after delivery per MD order; instruct in birth control measures to prevent pregnancy for one year after evacuation; encourage verbalization of feelings and provide emotional support.
Special Consideration: Human chorionic gonadotropin (HCG) levels are monitored for one year after evacuation for detection of choriocarcinoma.

HYPEREMESIS GRAVIDARUM

. . . .

INCOMPETENT CERVIX

. . . .

PLACENTA PREVIA

Definition: Intractable nausea and vomiting during pregnancy.
Causes: Unknown. May be related to psychological factors in some women.
Assessment Findings: Intractable nausea and vomiting; weight loss, s/s dehydration; fluid and electrolyte imbalance; confusion; rapid pulse; fruity breath; ketonuria and proteinuria.
Nursing Interventions: Monitor vital signs, I&O, weight, and calorie count; measures to alleviate nausea including medication such as Zofran if ordered; IV administration of fluids and electrolytes; NPO until no vomiting for 24 hours. Client education relating to resumption of oral intake: eating small frequent meals of low-fat, easily digested carbohydrates, eating in a sitting position and remaining in sitting position 30 minutes after meals, and taking liquids between meals versus with meals.
Special Consideration: Once vomiting stops and electrolyte balance is restored, pregnancy usually continues without recurrence.

• •

Definition: Premature dilation of cervix.
Causes: Cervical defects in structure or function.
Assessment Findings: Dilation of cervix (usually in 4th or 5th month); vaginal bleeding.
Nursing Interventions: Monitor vital signs and fetal heart rate; prepare client for cervical cerclage; postsurgical teaching: avoid intercourse, prolonged standing, heavy lifting; instruct client to report vaginal bleeding or increased uterine contractions to healthcare provider.
Special Consideration: Cervical cerclage removed at 37 weeks to allow for normal dilation of cervix in preparation of delivery.

• •

Definition: Placenta located over or near internal os. Three types exist: *Complete:* Completely covers internal os. *Partial:* partially covers internal os. *Marginal:* Margin of placenta overlaps with internal os.
Causes: Exact cause not known. Risk factors include advanced maternal age, previous uterine surgery, multiple pregnancy, or multiparity.
Assessment Findings: Painless bright red vaginal bleeding; previa depicted on ultrasound.
Nursing Interventions: Assess vital signs and fetal heart rate; evaluate bleeding, uterine tone, and contractibility; assess for hemorrhage; have oxygen available in case of fetal distress; initiate bed rest; if needed, prepare client for cesarean delivery, and administer betamethasone if fetus is premature. If bleeding ceases and client is to return home, obtain home-care referral. Encourage verbalization of feelings and provide emotional support.
Special Considerations: Monitor for postpartum hemorrhage due to decreased contractibility of uterus. Do NOT perform vaginal exam.

PREECLAMPSIA

. . . .

PRETERM LABOR

. . . .

PART
III

Definition: One type of gestational hypertension.

Causes: Exact cause not known; occurs more commonly in nulliparous women.

Assessment Findings: *Preeclampsia:* BP ≥140/90, proteinuria of 1 g in 24 hours, edema, weight gain >1 lb per week. *Severe preeclampsia:* BP ≥160/110, proteinuria of 5 g in 24 hours, severe edema, oiguira (400 mL or less in 24 hours), headaches, epigastric pain, hyperreflexia, visual disturbances.

Nursing Interventions: *Home management:* Instruct patient on monitoring BP, fetal movement count; teach medication regime (if prescribed), frequent rest periods or bed rest (if prescribed) and reporting of worsening symptoms. *Acute care:* Monitor vital signs and urinary output, edema, fetal heart tones, contractions; assess reflexes and for s/s seizure activity and convulsions; initiate seizure precautions; bed rest; limit visitors; medication administration as ordered (antihypertensives, magnesium sulfate).

· ·

Definition: Labor that occurs after 20 weeks gestation but before 37 weeks gestation.

Causes: Increased risk with placenta previa, incompetent cervix, premature rupture of membranes (PROM), urinary tract infection, preeclampsia, eclampsia, larger fetal size, multiple pregnancy, fetal death.

Assessment Findings: Uterine contractions every 10 min. for 2 hours despite position change, lower abdominal cramping, dull low-back pain, pelvic pressure extending to back and thighs.

Nursing Interventions: Monitor vital signs, uterine contractions, fetal heart rate; bed rest in left lateral lying position; administer IV fluids per order; administer tocolytics per MD order; administer betamethasone if ordered; provide emotional support.

Special Considerations: Teach ALL pregnant women s/s preterm labor and to promptly report any s/s of preterm labor to their healthcare provider.

· ·

AMNIOTIC FLUID EMBOLISM

. . . .

DYSTOCIA

. . . .

FETAL DISTRESS

Definition: Amniotic fluid enters into maternal circulation.

Causes: Open venous sinus at placenta site; risk factors include premature rupture of membranes (PROM) and precipitous labor.

Assessment Findings: Acute onset of respiratory distress, chest pain, hypotension, cyanosis, seizure activity, hemorrhage, hypoxia, fetal brady-cardia, fetal distress.

Nursing Interventions: Emergency measures to maintain life; position client on left side; monitor fetal status, administer IV fluids, blood products and medications per order; prepare for emergency delivery when client stabilizes; provide emotional support to client/family.

Special Consideration: Amniotic fluid embolism has a high fatality rate.

• •

Definition: Difficult, prolonged labor.

Causes: Fetus that is large, malpositioned, or with abnormal presentation; hypotonic contractions (irregular and weak) or hypertonic (painful, fre-quent, and uncoordinated); cephalopelvic disproportion (CPD).

Assessment Findings: Abdominal pain, abnormal contraction pattern, lack of progression of labor, maternal fatigue, maternal tachycardia, fetal distress.

Nursing Interventions: Monitor vital signs, contractions, fetal heart rate; assist with pelvic exam and ultrasound (if ordered); administer IV fluids as prescribed; administer oxytocin as ordered; instruct client in relaxation and breathing techniques; monitor color of amniotic fluid; administer pain medication and sedatives as ordered.

Special Consideration: The condition is addressed by treating the underly-ing reason for the dystocia.

• •

Definition: Fetus not tolerating uterine environment.

Causes: Risk factors include preeclampsia, eclampsia, diabetes, Rh incom-patibility, prolapsed cord, factors interfering with functioning of placenta, postterm gestation, hypertonic uterine contractions, dystocia.

Assessment Findings: Fetal heart rate <120 or >160, meconium-stained amniotic fluid, variable decelerations and late decelerations, fetal hyperactivity.

Nursing Interventions: Stop oxytocin if being used; place client in left lateral side lying position; administer oxygen; notify physician; prepare for cesarean section.

FETAL DEMISE

. . . .

INVERTED UTERUS

PART
III

. . . .

PRECIPITATE LABOR

Definition: Fetal death.
Causes: Intrauterine environment not conducive to fetal health; fetal abnormalities.
Assessment Findings: Absent fetal movement; absent fetal heart tones.
Nursing Interventions: Encourage client/family to verbalize feelings, and offer support; support client/family religious and cultural practices, including labor and delivery; encourage family to hold infant, take pictures, make memory box.
Special Considerations: Utilize appropriate verbal and nonverbal communication techniques. Do not use clichés, such as "You can always have more," "It is better this way," and "I know how you feel."

. . . .

Definition: The uterus turns inside out during delivery of the placenta. It is also known as uterine inversion.
Cause: The placenta fails to detach from the uterus, pulling the uterus inside out as it is expelled.
Assessment Findings: Severe pain, hemorrhage, s/s shock; uterus may be seen protruding through the vagina.
Nursing Interventions: Assist with treatment for shock; monitor vital signs, monitor for hemorrhage.
Special Consideration: Uterus will be returned to correct position either through the vagina or through laparotomy.

. . . .

Definition: Rapid labor that lasts <3 hours.
Causes: Risk factors include previous labor of short duration.
Assessment Findings: Sudden, intense urge to push, bulging of the perineum, increase in bloody show, rupture of the membranes, crowning of the fetal head.
Nursing Interventions: Call for help, stay with client, offer emotional support, have client pant between contractions; do not attempt to stop delivery. If healthcare provider is not available, deliver baby as follows: Put on sterile gloves if available, support fetal head with one hand and apply gentle pressure to head, deliver between contractions ensuring cord is not wrapped around neck, use slight downward pressure to move anterior shoulder under pubic symphysis, suction mouth, hold infant level with placenta until cord is clamped; dry infant and place infant on mother's abdomen; allow placenta to separate and deliver placenta.
Special Considerations: If infant is delivered before physician arrives, check infant to be sure that it is breathing, and monitor mother closely for hemorrhage.

PREMATURE RUPTURE OF MEMBRANES (PROM)

. . . .

UTERINE RUPTURE

. . . .

Definition: Spontaneous rupture of the membranes before onset of regular contractions.

Causes: Risk factors include lack of prenatal care, poor nutrition, smoking, multiple gestations, uterine infection, incompetent cervix.

Assessment Findings: Blood-tinged amniotic fluid gushing or leaking from vagina.

Nursing Interventions: Verify drainage is amniotic fluid (nitrazine paper turns blue or amniotic fluid placed on a slide dries into a fernlike pattern); monitor for onset of contractions, monitor fetal well-being, monitor for s/s infection: maternal fever, tachycardia, increased white blood cells.

Special Consideration: In term pregnancy, if labor does not start within 24 hours, prepare to induce labor.

. . . .

Definition: Full-thickness separation of the uterine wall and the overlying serosa.

Causes: Stress on uterus exceeds its ability to stretch. Risk factors include multifetal gestation, large baby, previous cesarean section, fetal malpresentation, tetanic contractions, malapplication of forceps.

Assessment Findings: *Complete:* Sudden, sharp abdominal pain, cessation of contractions, vaginal bleeding, s/s shock, absent fetal heart tones. *Incomplete:* Localized tenderness, persistent aching pain, vital signs, fetal heart tones, and lack of contractions gradually point to maternal and fetal distress.

Nursing Interventions: Report immediately and prepare for immediate cesarean section; oxygen via mask; stat blood type and cross match, establish IV line and administer medications, fluids, and blood products as ordered; insert indwelling catheter; encourage verbalization of fears and provide emotional support.

. . . .

MASTITIS

- -

POSTPARTUM DEPRESSION

- -

POSTPARTUM HEMORRHAGE

Definition: Inflammation of the mammary glands.
Causes: Cracks or fissures on the nipples allow organisms from infant's mouth or nose or mother's unwashed hands to enter breast tissue.
Assessment Findings: Localized, reddened, swollen, painful area on breast that is warm to touch; fever, chills, flulike symptoms.
Nursing Interventions: Instruct client in good hand and breast hygiene; continue lactation in breast-feeding mothers—encourage proper latching on and removal of infant from breast; teach mother application of heat or cold to breast as ordered and medication regime.
Special Considerations: Teach all mothers proper infant latching on and removal from breast as well as proper breast and hand hygiene to prevent mastitis.

· ·

Definition: A prolonged and intense feeling of sadness and/or hopelessness that occurs within one year after giving birth.
Causes: A combination of physical, emotional, and lifestyle factors.
Assessment Findings: Intense feeling of sadness or hopelessness; crying; difficulty concentrating; loss of pleasure in daily activities; weight changes, sleeplessness, fatigue, decreased energy level, feelings of guilt or worthlessness, anxiety, agitation, thoughts of suicide.
Nursing Interventions: Monitor bonding with infant, appropriate infant development, suicide risk; teach/encourage compliance with treatment regime, including medications (Prozac, Zoloft, Paxil); encourage verbalization of feelings.
Special Considerations: Teach all mothers s/s postpartum depression and to seek treatment. Assess all postpartum clients for depression throughout the postpartum period.

· ·

Definition: Loss of 500 mL of blood after vaginal delivery or 1,000 mL of blood after a cesarean section within a 24-hour period. *Early postpartum hemorrhage:* Occurs in first 24 hours after delivery. *Late postpartum hemorrhage:* Occurs 24 hours to 6 weeks after delivery.
Causes: Uterine atony; retained placenta, vaginal lacerations, DIC.
Assessment Findings: Bleeding from vagina: can be sudden gush or prolonged seepage; with sufficient blood loss will exhibit s/s hypovolemic shock (restlessness, dizziness, lightheadedness, increased pulse, narrowing pulse pressure, pallor, decreased urinary output).
Nursing Interventions: If uterine is soft and/or boggy, massage uterus; notify physician; monitor vital signs, blood loss via peri pad count, level of consciousness, hematocrit and hemoglobin; administer IV fluid, blood products, and/or oxytocin as ordered.
Special Consideration: Uterine atony is the number one cause of postpartum hemorrhage.

PUERPERAL INFECTION

. . . .

UTERINE ATONY

. . . .

Definition: Infection of the birth canal and other structures during the postpartum period.

Causes: Presence of microbes along with predisposing factors such as prolonged/difficult labor, PROM, cesarean section, frequent or unsanitary vaginal examinations, retain placenta, hemorrhage, episiotomy or lacerations.

Assessment Findings: Temperature of 102°F that lasts for two consecutive days, chills, headache, malaise, restlessness, anxiety.

Nursing Interventions: Monitor vital signs, I&O, drainage; encourage bed rest, frequent voiding; teach/encourage frequent peri pad changes and proper perineal hygiene; administer antibiotics and analgesics as per order.

Special Considerations: Whether or not mother can continue to breast-feed is dependent on the antibiotic being administered and the overall condition of the mother.

· ·

Definition: Failure of myometrium of the uterus to contract.

Causes: Risk factors include multiple gestations, injury to birth canal, magnesium use during labor, rapid delivery, delivery with forceps or vacuum assisted, retained placenta fragments, dystocia, endometritis.

Assessment Findings: Soft or boggy uterus.

Nursing Interventions: Gently message uterus; if ineffective, notify physician; administer oxytocin if ordered.

Special Considerations: Normally, contraction of the myometrium of the uterus compresses blood vessels in the uterus to prevent bleeding. If left untreated, uterine atony can lead to postpartum hemorrhage.

· ·

ANTENATAL CORTICOSTEROIDS

. . . .

ERGOT ALKALOIDS

. . . .

MAGNESIUM SULFATE

Example Medications	Betamethasone, Celestone, dexamethasone.
Uses	Used when preterm delivery is imminent to increase production of fetal surfactant in order to accelerate maturation of fetal lungs and subsequent incidence of respiratory distress syndrome (RSD) in the preterm infant.
Adverse Reactions	Suppression of maternal immune system; pulmonary edema; elevated blood sugar in women with diabetes.
Nursing Interventions	Administered IM in repeated doses (once every 24 hours × 2 or every 12 hours × 4, depending on medication given).
Special Consideration	Labor must be stopped long enough for repeated doses of the corticosteroid to be administered and produce desired effect.

· ·

Example Medications	Methergine, Ergotrate Maleate.
Uses	Postpartum hemorrhage.
Adverse Reactions	GI: Nausea. CP: Bradycardia, arrhythmias, severe hypertension, myocardial infarction, respiratory depression. GU: Uterine cramping, tetany. Neuro: Confusion, seizures.
Nursing Interventions	Close monitoring of blood pressure—if BP elevated, hold medication and notify physician.
Special Consideration	Contraindicated during pregnancy and in clients with cardiovascular disease.

· ·

Category	Central nervous system depressant and anticonvulsant.
Use	Prevent/stop preterm labor. Prevent/control seizures in women with preeclampsia and eclampsia.
Adverse Reactions	Toxicity in the newborn. Depression of reflexes, respiration. Decreased urinary output. Hypotension. Pulmonary edema.
Nursing Interventions	Monitor closely for signs of toxicity: suppressed patellar reflex, respiratory rate <12/min., urinary output less than 30 mL/hour.
Special Considerations	Keep antidote (calcium gluconate) readily available. Stop infusion 2 hours before delivery. Often administered in the first 24–48 hours postpartum for women with preeclampsia or eclampsia.

OPIOIDS

. . . .

PROSTAGLANDINS

. . . .

RhoGAM

Example Medications	Dilaudid, Phenergan, Sublimaze, Stadol, Nubain.
Uses	Relieve labor pain.
Adverse Reactions	Dizziness; nausea and vomiting. Decreased blood pressure, respirations. Sedation, somnolence, seizures, stupor, coma. Diaphoresis, confusion.
Nursing Interventions	Obtain drug history; do not use if history of opiod dependency. Monitor respirations and hold medication if <12/min. Monitor fetal heart rate.
Special Consideration	Keep antidote, Narcan, readily available.

. . . .

Example Medications	Prostaglandin E, Cervidil, Perpidil, Dinoprostone.
Uses	Ripening of cervix for labor induction. Labor induction.
Adverse Reactions	Nausea, diarrhea, stomach cramps. Hyperstimulation of uterus. Fetal distress. Headache, hypotension, fever, chills.
Nursing Interventions	Have client void prior to administration. Keep client in supine or lateral position after administration (30–60 min. gel; 2 hours vaginal insert).
Special Consideration	Oxytocin can be administered 6 to 12 hours after cessation of prostiglandin.

. . . .

Category	Immune globulin.
Use	Prevent isoimmunization in Rh-negative clients with potential/ actual exposure to fetal Rh-positive blood.
Adverse Reactions	Elevated temperature.
Nursing Interventions	Administer IM (usual dose 300 micrograms). Administer at 28 weeks' gestation and within 72 hours of delivery.
Special Consideration	Not effective once client develops positive antibody titer.

TOCOLYTICS

. . . .

UTERINE STIMULANTS

. . . .

Example Medications	Indocin, nifedipine, terbutaline.
Use	Stop uterine contractions and prevent preterm delivery.
Adverse Reactions	Depends on specific medication.
Nursing Interventions	Have client assume lateral position to decrease cervical pressure. Monitor vital signs, fetal well-being, contractions, dilation, urinary output. Provide support to client and family.
Special Considerations	Do not use in women with severe preeclampsia or eclampsia when gestational age >37 weeks or cervical dilation is >4 cm.

. . . .

Example Medications	Pitocin, oxytocin.
Uses	Induction or augmentation of labor. Postpartum hemorrhage.
Adverse Reactions	Uterine hypertonicity/rupture. Hypotension followed by rebound hypertension. Arrhythmias.
Nursing Interventions	Monitor blood pressure, contractions, fetal heart rate closely. Administer IV with additive piggybacked at port closest to IV insertion site.
Special Consideration	Monitor closely for postpartum hemorrhage, as uterus may become soft or boggy when uterine stimulant wears off.

MONTH 1

. . . .

MONTH 2

PART
III

. . . .

MONTH 3

Fertilization/Conception	Egg (23 chromosomes) and sperm (23 chromosomes) unite, creating zygote (46 chromosomes or 23 pairs).
Zygote	Undergoes rapid cell division and becomes a mass of cells called a blastocyte.
Blastocyte	Travels through fallopian tubes and implants into uterus 7 to 10 days after fertilization and is called an embryo.
Embryo	By end of the month is the size of a grain of rice.

. . . .

Embryo	Divides into three layers: *Ectoderm:* Develops into brain, nerves, skin, hair, nails, tooth enamel. *Mesoderm:* Develops into bones, muscles, blood, heart, kidneys, reproductive system, part of lungs. *Endoderm:* Develops into other part of lungs, liver, intestines, urinary tract.
Week 5	Embryo forms two grooves. One end becomes the head, while the other becomes the tail.
Weeks 6–8	Head differentiates from tail. Bumps mark arms and legs. Tiny hands and feet start to develop. Heart develops and starts to beat. Tongue, teeth, and eyelids start to form. Umbilical cord developed.
Fetus	Called a fetus from 8 weeks until end of pregnancy.

. . . .

Developmental Milestones	Fetal heart rate can be detected with Doppler. Body uncurls from "C" position. Tail disappears. Reproductive system forming. Eyelids, earlobes, limbs, digits continue to form.
Weight	1 ounce.
Length	3 inches.

MONTH 4

. . . .

MONTH 5

. . . .

MONTH 6

Developmental Milestones	Fetus can hear. Major organs complete but not functional. Swallows, kicks, may do somersaults.
Weight	6 ounces.
Length	7 inches.

· ·

Developmental Milestones	Mother may experience quickening (baby's movements). Lanugo develops. Vernix caseosa develops. Sucks thumb. Meconium forming.
Weight	10 to 16 ounces.
Length	7 to 10 inches.

· ·

Developmental Milestones	Heartbeat heard with stethoscope. Essential organs fully formed. Bones become harder. Reacts to noises. Facial features more recognizable.
Weight	1.5 to 2 pounds.
Length	10 to 13 inches.

MONTH 7

. . . .

MONTH 8

PART
III

. . . .

MONTH 9

Developmental Milestones	Brain sections form for distinct functions. Taste buds develop. Protective fat begins to develop. Able to blink. Eyes remain open for short periods of time. Testicles move to groin (in males).
Weight	2.5 to 3.5 pounds.
Length	11 to 16 inches.

Developmental Milestones	Brain develops rapidly. All organs except lungs mature. Skin starts to smoothen. Fingernails grow past fingertips. Limited room for movement—settles into head-down position.
Weight	4 to 6 pounds.
Length	16 to 18 inches from head to toe.

Developmental Milestones	Lungs mature. Assumes birth position—lightening may occur. Fat layers thicken. Vernix caseosa and lanugo begin to disappear. Labor begins.
Weight	6 to 8 pounds on average.
Length	20 to 22 inches on average.

FETAL CIRCULATION

· ·

Urotoplacental Circulation	Brings oxygen-rich blood from mother to intervillious spaces via uterine arteries and then back to maternal circulation via veins.
Fetoplacental Circulation	Oxygen-depleted blood from fetus transported by umbilical arteries and oxygen-rich blood returned to fetus via umbilical vein.
Foramen Ovale	Shunts fetal blood from right atrium to left atrium, bypassing lungs.
Ductus Arteriosis	Shunts fetal blood from pulmonary artery to aorta.
Fetal Circulatory Path	Oxygen-rich blood from umbilical vein to fetal inferior vena cava. Right atrium to foramen ovale to left atrium to left ventricle to aorta. Some blood from right atrium goes to right ventricle to pulmonary artery to ductus arteriosis to aorta. Oxygen-depleted blood to umbilical arteries.

FETAL HEART RATE ACCELERATION

. . . .

FETAL HEART RATE: EARLY DECELERATION

. . . .

FETAL HEART RATE: LATE DECELERATION

PART III

Fetal accelerations are a healthy response to fetal movement. They are considered a reassuring sign in the fetus.

• •

Definition: Slowing of the fetal heart rate (FHR) that occurs in conjunction with maternal contractions.
Causes: Compression of fetal head during labor.
Assessment Findings: Slowing of FHR 20 to 30 beats per minute under baseline.
Nursing Interventions: Benign event; reassure patient that fetus is not at risk; continue to monitor and document FHR.
Special Consideration: May progress to variable deceleration.

• •

Definition: Decreased fetal heart rate in response to decreased blood flow during contractions or a structural defect in the placenta.
Nursing Interventions: Turn mother on left side; administer oxygen by mask, increase IV fluid rate per standing order; notify physician.

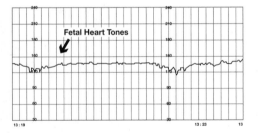

FETAL HEART RATE VARIABILITY

. . . .

FETAL HEART TONES

. . . .

FUNDAL HEIGHT

PART III

Definition: A fluctuation in heart rate that represents the interaction between the sympathetic and parasympathetic nervous systems. Interaction between the two systems results in changes in the fetal heart rate. Variability indicates that both systems are working.

. . . .

Third Month	Can be heard via Doppler.
Sixth Month	Can be heard via stethoscope.
Normal Rate	120 to 160 beats per minute.

. . . .

Definition: Measurement from the top of the maternal symphysis pubic notch to the top of the fundus in centimeters. According to McDonald's Rule, the measurement in centimeters will approximate the weeks of gestation. It is an indirect measurement of fetal growth.

NCLEX-RN Flash Review

LEOPOLD MANEUVERS

First Maneuver	Face mother's head. Palpate uterine fundus. Determine fetal body part at fundus.
Second Maneuver	Continue facing mother's head. Palpate with one hand on each side of fundus. Determine location of fetal spine and extremities.
Third Maneuver	Face mother's feet. Palpate above symphysis pubis. Determine fetal presenting part. Determine if fetal descent has occurred.
Fourth Maneuver	Continue facing mother's feet. Exert gentle downward pressure on fetal head. Palpate presenting part between thumb and forefinger. Determine if cephalic versus breech presentation.

ACROCYANOSIS

....

APGAR SCORE

....

CAPUT SUCCEDANEUM

Definition: Cyanosis of hands, feet, and perioral area in the newborn due to immature circulatory system. It is a common and benign finding in the newborn.

• •

Sign	0	1	2
Heart Rate	Absent	<100/min.	>100/min.
Respirations	Absent	Weak cry; hypoventilation	Strong cry
Muscle Tone	Flaccid	Some flexion	Active motion
Reflex Irritability	No response	Weak cry; grimace	Strong cry or withdrawal
Color	Pallor; cyanotic	Pink body with blue extremities	Completely pink

Evaluate at 1 and 5 minutes after birth.
Score of 8 to 10, no interventions required; 4 to 7, gentle stimulation, administer oxygen; 0 to 3 requires resuscitation measures.

• •

Definition: Edema of the soft tissue of the head that crosses over suture lines. It is a benign condition that resolves a few days after birth.

CEPHALHEMATOMA

. . . .

EPSTEIN PEARLS

. . . .

FONTANELS

PART
III

Definition: Swelling in the head between the bone and periosteum. It does not cross suture lines. It usually resolves in 6 weeks and requires no treatment.

• •

Definition: Small white or yellow benign lumps on the neonate's gums or hard palate. They are caused by retained secretions and resolve on their own.

• •

Definition: Soft spots located on the anterior and posterior portion of the fetal head that enable the head to mold in order to pass through the birth canal.

Anterior Fontanel	Diamond shape 3–4 cm Firm, flat Closed by end of 18 months
Posterior Fontanel	Triangular shape 0.5 to 1 cm Firm, flat Closed by end of second month
Bulging Fontanels	Increased intercranial pressure
Sunken Fontanels	Dehydration

HARLEQUIN COLOR CHANGES

. . . .

HEAD LAG

. . . .

HEAD TO TOE: HEENT/NEUROLOGICAL

Definition: A benign change in the neonate's skin color where one half of the neonate's skin turns dark pink or red and the other half turns pale. The division can be vertical as if a line is drawn from the center of the neonate's forehead to the pubis or horizontally as if a line was drawn across the abdomen. These color changes are due to the neonate's instability and the reactivity of its blood vessels.

. . . .

Definition: When infant is moving from lying to sitting position, head droops forward or backward. This is a normal occurrence due to lack of control/strength of the neck muscles. It should be nearly gone by 12 weeks and should completely disappear by 20 weeks. In its most severe form, it may occur in infants with Down syndrome, brain damage, and/or hypoxia.

. . . .

Head	Fontanels soft. Able to turn head to side if placed on same surface. Head lag.
Eyes	Blue or slate gray—permanent eye color established at 3 to 12 months. Tearless crying. Doll's eyes normal for first 10 days.
Ears	Pina flat against side of head. Top of ear parallel or above inner canthus of eye.
Nose	Obligatory nose breathers.
Throat and Mouth	No cleft in palate. Scant saliva. Pink lips.
Neurological	Reflexes present and not hypo/hyperreflexive.

HEAD TO TOE: HEAD-TO-CHEST RATIO

. . . .

HEAD TO TOE: HEART AND LUNGS

PART III

. . . .

HEAD TO TOE: ABDOMEN/GENITALIA/
SPINE/EXTREMITIES

Definition: The circumference of the neonate's head compared to the circumference of the chest; the head circumference should be 1 to 3 cm greater than that of the chest. If the head circumference is greater than 3 cm larger than the chest circumference, increased intercranial pressure or hydrocephaly might be indicated. Head circumference less than 1 cm larger than the chest circumference can be indicative of molding, anencephaly, and/or closed suture lines.

. . . .

Heart Rate	110–160/min.
Heart Sounds	Murmurs are common, but every murmur should be referred to physician for further evaluation.
Apical Impulse (point of maximal impulse)	4th intercostal space.
Respiratory Rate	30–50/min. Slight retractions are normal.
Abdominal	Neonates are abdominal versus chest breathers.

. . . .

Abdomen	Cylindrical in shape. Bowel sounds present few hours after birth. Umbilical cord white and gelatin-like—begins to dry within 1–2 hours after delivery. Umbilical cord with two arteries and one vein. Liver palpable 1 inch below costal margin.
Genitalia	*Male:* Testes descended; urinary meatus at penile tip; scrotal edema may be present for first few days after birth. *Female:* Vaginal discharge may be present.
Spine	Straight and intact. No dimpling or hair tufts.
Extremities	Bowlegged and flat feet. Polydactyl and/or syndactyl not present. Acrocyanosis may be present. Extremities in flexed position.

LANUGO

. . . .

MECONIUM

. . . .

MILIA

Definition: Fine, downy hair that develops during the 5th month of gestation to protect the fetal skin. It begins to disappear during the 9th month of gestation. It is considered normal for the infant to be born with some remaining, and it will disappear on its own. The amount with which the infant is born depends on the length of gestation: greater gestational age equates to a lesser amount.

· ·

Definition: The first stool passed by the neonate. It is tarry in consistency and black or dark green in color. When meconium is noted in the amniotic fluid, it is considered a sign of fetal distress and can lead to respiratory difficulties in the neonate.

· ·

Definition: Small white bumps appearing over neonate's nose, chin, and/ or cheeks. These are due to sebaceous glands being clogged. They are considered benign and will disappear on their own.

MOLDING

....

MONGOLIAN SPOTS

....

REFLEXES

Definition: Oblong shape of the neonate head caused by pressure on the head as it passes through the birth canal. This occurs due to the cranial suture lines and fontanels allowing the cranial plates to move during the birthing process to narrow the diameter of the head to facilitate the birthing process.

. . . .

Definition: Blue to slate gray marks on the neonate's buttocks, back, and legs that resemble bruises. They are a benign color variation and are more prevalent in Native American, African American, Asian, and Hispanic neonates. They usually disappear by age 2.

. . . .

Babinski	Toes fan upward.
Grasping	Neonate grasps healthcare provider's finger when placed in palm.
Moro/Startle	When neonate is lowered suddenly or startled by a loud noise, neonate extends arms and legs and then abducts them.
Rooting	When side of check is brushed gently, neonate turns head and opens mouth.
Stepping	Neonate moves feet in a stepping motion when held upright with soles of feet touching flat surface.
Suck	When nipple, pacifier, or clean gloved finger is placed in neonate's mouth, neonate begins to suck.
Tonic Neck/Fencing	When neonate's head is turned to one side, neonate extends arm on that side and flexes opposite arm.

VERNIX CASEOSA

Definition: White cheesy substance that forms a protective coating over the fetal skin. It develops during the 5th gestational month and begins to disappear during the 9th month. The amount remaining at birth is dependent on gestational age. It is considered a normal finding.

· ·

BREAST-FEEDING TIPS

. . . .

CIRCUMCISION CARE

. . . .

UMBILICAL CORD

Latching On	Brush infant's lower lip with nipple. When infant opens his or her mouth widely, guide nipple and areola into mouth.
Release	Insert a clean finger into side of infant's mouth to release suction. Remove nipple and areola from mouth.
Hygiene	Wash daily with warm water. Do not use soap on the nipples, as this may lead to cracking; may express a few drops of breast milk and apply to nipples to prevent dryness.
Sore/Cracked Nipples	Ensure infant is latching on correctly. Rotate position of infant each feeding. Cracked nipples: expose to air 20 min. after each feeding.
Engorgement	Breast-feed frequently. Apply warm, moist heat 20 minutes before each feeding. Apply ice between feedings for 20 minutes.
Caloric Needs	Mother should increase calories by 200 to 500 daily.

Nursing interventions first 24 hours after circumcision	Check for bleeding; if bleeding occurs, apply pressure with sterile gauze. Allow first dressing to fall off naturally. Apply diapers loosely. Monitor urination. Do not place neonate with petroleum dressing under radiant warmer due to risk for burns.
Teach parents daily care	Cleanse with warm water; do not use baby wipes due to alcohol content. Apply petroleum jelly or antimicrobial ointment (per hospital policy). Change diapers every 4 hours. Notify practitioner if redness, swelling, or discharge is present.

Arteries/Vein	There should be 2 arteries and 1 vein.
Clamping	Keep cord clamped for first 24 hours after birth.
Daily Care	Varies by hospital policy/protocol but may include cleansing around cord and application of drying agent or antimicrobial agent.
Infection	Parents should be taught to monitor for and report signs of infection including moistness, oozing, discharge, redness around insertion site.
Falling Off	Cord shrivels and dries and eventually falls off in approximately 7 to 10 days.

DRUG-DEPENDENT NEONATE

FETAL ALCOHOL SYNDROME

PART
III

HYPERBILIRUBINEMIA

Definition: Infant dependent on the drug mother used during pregnancy.
Cause: Repeated intrauterine absorption of drug from maternal blood.
Assessment Findings: Depends on amount and type of drug used by mother but includes irritability, hyperactivity, tremors, exaggerated reflexes, difficult to console, sweating, acrocyanosis, convulsions, respiratory distress, hunger, mental retardation, developmental delays.
Nursing Interventions: Position lying on side, head dependent position; suction excess secretions with bulb syringe; decrease environmental stimuli; collect urine for toxicology studies; mitts on hands; administer medications such as morphine sulfate, methadone, or phenobarbital as ordered.

. . . .

Definition: Permanent damage experienced by fetus from exposure to maternal alcohol consumption.
Cause: Maternal alcohol consumption.
Assessment Findings: Epicanthal folds, small mandible and/or chin; long, thin upper lip; irritability, difficult to console; poor feeding; high-pitched cry.
Nursing Interventions: Reduce environmental stimuli; maintain hydration and nutrition; administer sedatives as ordered; provide emotional support to mother.

. . . .

Definition: Yellow discoloration of the skin due to excess bilirubin in the neonate's blood.
Causes: Immaturity of the neonate's liver makes it slow to process the by-product of red blood cell breakdown, bilirubin, leading to buildup of bilirubin in the blood.
Assessment Findings: Yellow discoloration of the skin that starts at the face and moves down to the chest and then legs. *Physiological jaundice:* Starts the 3rd or 4th day of life and resolves by the 7th day. Bilirubin levels do not exceed 12 mg/dl. *Pathological jaundice:* Starts within first 24 hours of life. Bilirubin levels exceed 17 mg/dl.
Nursing Interventions: Monitor jaundice and bilirubin levels. Maintain feedings and offer extra feedings or water to neonate; teach/administer phototherapy as ordered; reassure parents.
Special Consideration: Neonate's stool may appear green due to excreted bile.

HYPOGLYCEMIA

. . . .

MECONIUM ASPIRATION

. . . .

PRETERM NEONATE

Definition: Glucose level <40mg/dL in full-term infant and <45 mg/dl in preterm infant.

Cause: Loss of maternal glucose supply; risk increased for infants of diabetic mothers; preterm and postterm infants; infants small for gestational age; and infants of mothers with preeclampsia.

Assessment Findings: Sweating, unstable temperature, high-pitched and shrill cry, tachypnea, jitteriness, lethargy, tremors, convulsions.

Nursing Interventions: Administer oral or intravenous glucose as per order.

Special Consideration: Monitor for rebound effect after administration of glucose.

. . . .

Definition: Resultant blockage of the neonate's airway from inhaling meconium mixed into the amniotic fluid.

Cause: Fetal distress during labor.

Assessment Findings: Meconium-stained amniotic fluid; cyanosis, limpness, increased respiratory effort, apnea, grunting, tachypnea, low Apgar score; course crackling lung sounds.

Treatment: Suction nose and mouth as soon as head is delivered; tracheal suctioning may be needed; chest therapy; antibiotics.

Special Considerations: Meconium aspiration may lead to aspiration pneumonia, cerebral palsy, mental retardation, seizures, pneumothorax.

. . . .

Definition	Neonate born before 37 weeks' gestation
Risk Factors	Multiple pregnancy, adolescent pregnancy, low socioeconomic status, lack of prenatal care, smoking, substance abuse, cervical incompetence, PROM, placenta previa, preeclampsia, eclampsia
Complications	Respiratory distress syndrome, intraventricular hemorrhage, retinopathy of prematurity, patent ductus arteriosus, necrotizing enterocolitis, apnea of prematurity

RESPIRATORY DISTRESS SYNDROME

. . . .

Definition: A lung disorder that primarily affects premature infants.
Causes: Insufficient production of pulmonary surfactant to coat the aveoli in order to keep them open for gas exchange. The aveoli close, leading to atelectasis, increased effort to breathe. Risk factors include premature birth, fetal hypoxia, and maternal diabetes.
Assessment Findings: Increased respiratory rate and effort, retractions, crackles on auscultation, nasal flaring, cyanosis, tachypnea, expiratory grunt.
Nursing Interventions: Ensure adequate thermoregulation; provide warmed, humidified oxygen via hood, nasal prongs, continuous positive airway pressure, or mechanical ventilation per order; suction when necessary with bulb syringe; provide emotional support for parents.
Special Consideration: Assess and treat for respiratory and metabolic acidosis.

. . . .

EYE PROPHYLAXIS

....

LUNG SURFACTANTS

....

LUNG SURFACTANTS

Example Medications/ Ointments	Erythromycin 0.5%, tetraclycine 1%, silver nitrate 1%.
Use	Protection from *N. gonorrhoeae* and *C. trachomatis*.
Adverse Reactions	Chemical conjunctivitis.
Nursing Implications	Administer within one hour of birth.
Special Considerations	Administration required by law.

• •

Example Medications	Beractant, calfactant, poractant alfa.
Use	Prevention/treatment of respiratory distress syndrome (RDS) in neonates.
Adverse Reactions	Bradycardia, oxygen desaturation, pulmonary hemorrhage, mucous plug.
Nursing Implications	Administer via endotrachial tube. Do not suction for 2 hours after medication administration.

• •

Part **IV**

PEDIATRICS, GENERAL

DEVELOPMENTAL PERIODS

. . . .

DIRECTION OF GROWTH

. . . .

THEORISTS: ERIK ERIKSON

Prenatal	Conception to birth
Infancy	0–12 months
Toddler	1–3 years
Preschooler	3–5 years
Elementary School Age	6–10 years
Adolescent	11–18 years
Young Adult	19–35 years
Middle Adult	36–64 years
Older Adult	65 and over

| Cephalocaudal | Growth proceeds from the head down to feet. Example: Head grows more than body during first 5 months' gestation. |
| Proximodistal | Growth occurs from the center of the body outward. Example: Infant gains control of arm movements, then finger movements. |

Infant	Trust versus mistrust
Toddler	Autonomy versus shame and doubt
Preschooler	Initiative versus guilt
Elementary School Age	Industry versus inferiority
Adolescent	Identity versus role confusion
Young Adult	Intimacy versus isolation
Middle Adult	Generativity versus stagnation
Older Adult	Integrity versus despair

THEORISTS: SIGMUND FREUD

. . . .

THEORISTS: LAWRENCE KOHLBERG

PART
IV

. . . .

THEORISTS: JEAN PIAGET

Age	Stage
0–1 Year	Oral sensory: Focus is on mouth and need to suck.
1–3 Years	Anal-urethra: Focus is on learning to control bowels.
3–6 Years	Phallic-locomotion: Self-centered attention; identifies with parent of opposite sex; superego develops.
6–12 Years	Latency: suppresses sexual desires to focus on skill achievement.
13–18 Years	Genitality: seeks mature sexual pleasure with partner.

Age	Stage/Phase
0–3 Years	Preconventional: Punishment and obedience orientation.
3–6 Years	Preconventional: Self-interest orientation.
6–12 Years	Conventional: Good-boy, nice-girl orientation; law-and-order orientation.
13+ Years	Postconventional: Social contract orientation; universal ethical principle orientation.

Age	Levels of Development
0–2 Years	Sensorimotor: Understands cause and effect; understands object permanence; understands night and day.
2–7 Years	Preoperational thought: Attributes life to inanimate objects; sees self as center of the world; understands only one piece of information at a time; uses pretend play; follows rules.
7–12 Years	Concrete operational thought: Understands more than one piece of information at a time; focus is on present; realistic understanding of world.
12+ Years	Formal operational thought: Thinks abstractly; cultural practices help child develop rules and develop sense of what is right or wrong.

INFANT: FINE/GROSS MOTOR

· ·

INFANT: LANGUAGE/COGNITIVE/SOCIAL

PART
IV

· ·

TODDLER: FINE/GROSS MOTOR

Age	Fine Motor	Gross Motor
0–3 Months	Hands open and at midline.	Lifts self up on forearms from prone position.
4–6 Months	Transfers objects from one hand to the other.	Rolls from back to front; supports weight on extended arms.
7–9 Months	Pincer grasp.	Sits independently.
10–12 Months	Takes objects out of container; scribbles	Pulls to standing position.

· ·

	Language	Cognitive	Social
0–3 Months	Orients to voice; smiles.	Regards toys.	Social smile; recognizes mother.
4–6 Months	Vocalizes pleasure and displeasure.	Focuses on action of object; searches briefly for toy moved out of sight.	Discriminates strangers.
7–9 Months	Babbles; nonspecific "mama" and "dada."	Uncovers partially hidden toy; repeats actions to repeat consequences.	Smiles at mirror image; feeds self with fingers.
10–12 Months	Waves bye-bye; specific "dada" and "mama."	Plays peekaboo; shakes rattle for attention.	Increasing awareness of strangers.

· ·

Age	Fine Motor	Gross Motor
13–15 Months	Scribbles spontaneously; stacks 2 blocks; puts pegs in pegboard.	Walks alone; throws ball.
16–18 Months	Begins to work puzzles.	Stands, squats, and stoops.
19–24 Months	Stacks 6 blocks; imitates vertical pencil stroke.	Kicks large ball; walks up steps using nonalternating feet.
25–33 Months	Copies a circle; strings beads.	Jumps in place; walks on tiptoes.

TODDLER: LANGUAGE/COGNITIVE/SOCIAL

· ·

PRESCHOOLERS

· ·

PLAY

Age	Language	Cognitive	Social/Adaptive
13–15 Months	Follows one-step commands; verbalizes 2 to 6 words.	Pretend play emerges.	Cooperates with dressing; drinks well from cup.
16–18 Months	7 to 20 words; points to body parts.	Pretend and imaginative play.	Imitates household chores.
19–24 Months	Two-word combinations; points to pictures.	Symbolic use of materials—baby bed in a shoe box.	Uses fork; takes off coat.
25–33 Months	Understands the prepositions *on*, *under*, and/or *behind*.	Categorizes objects by color, shape, or function; counts.	Feeds self without a mess; bathes with assistance; puts on pants/shoes.

Age	Play	Language
3 Years	Solitary or parallel play; puppets, large ball, sand, and water; rides tricycle.	Vocabulary 900 to 2,000 words; knows first and last name; talks to self.
4 Years	Imaginative and dramatic play; imaginary playmates; dresses up; enjoys crayons, paints, books.	Vocabulary 1,500 to 3,000 words; uses "I"; asks questions; counts to 5.
5 Years	Realistic play; enjoys musical instruments; runs, jumps, rides bicycle; chooses friends with like interests.	Vocabulary of 2,100 to 5,000 words; repeats sentences of 12 or more syllables; can tell story accurately.

Type of Play	Age	Description
Solitary	Infant	Plays alone. Enjoys presence of others but is focused on own activity.
Parallel	Toddler	Plays alongside but not with others. Example: Two boys playing with trucks but no interaction with each other.
Associative	Preschooler	Plays together with others but no group goal.
Cooperative	School age	Follows organized rules; definite leader/follower relationship.

ABDOMEN/GENITALIA

. . . .

HEAD/EYES/EARS/NOSE/MOUTH

PART
IV

. . . .

MUSCULATURE

Abdomen	Prominent in standing and supine positions until the age of 4 years. Prominent when standing until puberty. Bowel sounds every 10 to 30 seconds. Use child's hand under yours during palpation if child is ticklish. Rigid abdomen almost always emergent problem.
Male Genitalia	Foreskin retracts. Urinary meatus at tip of glans penis. No discharge. Testes palpable in scrotum.
Female Genitalia	No vaginal discharge. Internal exam recommended ages 16 and over or when sexually active.

Head	Normocephalic; symmetrical

Eyes	Outer canthus aligns with tip of pinna.
	Epicanthal folds common in Asian children.
	Acuity: 1 year: 20/200
	           2 years: 20/70
	           5 years: 20/30
	           6 years: 20/20

Ears	Tympanic membrane intact, pearly gray color. (Gently pull pinna down and back for otoscopic exam.) Low-set ears suggest mental retardation.
Nose	Infants are nose breathers. Turbinates pink and without edema.
Mouth	Tonsils large—reach maximum between 10 and 12 years. No cleft in palate.

Motor Function	Hand preference develops around 4 years of age.
Gait	*Genu varum:* Bowlegged: ages 1–2 years. *Genu valgum:* Knock-kneed: ages 2–7 years.
Spine	Lumbar curve develops at 12–18 months. Newborns have flexed position.

NEUROLOGICAL: REFLEXES

. . . .

SKIN

. . . .

TEETH/CHEST/HEART/LUNGS

Reflex	Age Disappears
Stepping	2 months
Moro "Startle"	3 months
Rooting	3–4 months
Palmar Grasp	3–4 months
Tonic Neck "Fencing"	4–6 months
Plantar Grasp	8–10 months
Sucking	10–12 months
Babinski	Converts to adult response by 2 years.

- -

Normal Findings	Lesion-free, soft, warm, good turgor.
Café au Lait Spot	Light brown birthmark that is round or oval in shape; may appear at birth or first years of life; one is common but more than six can be indicative of neurocutaneous disease.
Hemangioma/ Strawberry	Birthmarks that are made up of increased blood vessels; appear red, blue, or purple in color; increase in size over first 8 months of life; eventually will fade/disappear but takes years.
Port-Wine Stain	Dark red or bluish birthmark that is usually large with irregular borders and occurs on the face and scalp; does not fade with time.

- -

Teeth	Begin to erupt at 4–6 months. All teeth erupted by 36 months. Begin losing baby teeth by ages 5–6.
Chest	Anterior-to-posterior ratio 1:2. Abdominal breathers under age of 7.
Lung Sounds	May have hyperresonance due to thin chest wall. Respiratory rate: 20–28 for ages 2–10 12–20 for ages 10–18
Heart Sounds	Innocent murmurs common. Sinus arrhythmia common. Apical impulse occurs in 4th intercostal space until age 7.

VACCINATION SCHEDULE, AGES 0 TO 6, FOR ALL (WITHOUT STIPULATIONS REGARDING HIGH-RISK STATUS)

. . . .

VACCINATION SCHEDULE, AGES 7 TO 18, FOR ALL (WITHOUT STIPULATIONS REGARDING HIGH-RISK STATUS)

PART
IV

. . . .

Age → Vaccine ↓	1 mo.	2 mos.	4 mos.	6 mos.	9 mos.	12 mos.	15 mos.	18 mos.	19–23 mos.	2–3 yrs.	4–6 yrs.
Hepatitis B	HepB 2nd dose[1]			HepB 3rd dose							
Rotavirus		RV	RV	RV (to 8 mos.)							
Diptheria, Tetanus, Pertussis		DTaP	DTaP	DTaP		see footnote 2.	DTaP				
Haemophilus influenza type b		Hib	Hib	Hib		Hib					
Inactivated Poliovirus		IPV	IPV	IPV							
Influenza				Influenza (yearly)							
Measles, Mumps, Rubella						MMR		See footnote 3.			MMR
Varicella						Varicella		See footnote 4.			
Hepatitis A						HepA (2 doses)					

1. First dose given at birth.
2. The fourth dose may be administered as early as age 12 months, provided at least 6 months have elapsed since the third dose.
3. The second dose may be administered before age 4 years, provided at least 4 weeks have elapsed since the first dose.
4. The second dose may be administered before age 4 years, provided at least 3 months have elapsed since the first dose.

Age → Vaccine ↓	7–10 yrs.	11–12 yrs.	13–18 yrs.
Diptheria, Tetanus, Pertussis	1 dose if indicated	1 dose	1 dose if indicated
Human papillomavirus	see footnote 1	3 doses	complete 3 does series
Meningococcal		MCV4	MCV4 catch-up immunization
Hepatitis B	Catch-up: Administer Hep B Series (3 doses)for those not previously vaccinated		
Inactivated Poliovirus	Catch-up: Administer IPV Series (3 doses) for those not previously vaccinated[2]		
Measles, Mumps, Rubella	Catch-up: Administer MMR Series (2 doses) for those not previously vaccinated[3]		
Varicella	Catch-up: Administer Varicella Series for (2 doses) those not previously vaccinated[4]		

1. The vaccine series can be started beginning at age 9 years; administer the second dose 1 to 2 months after the first dose and the third dose 6 months after the first dose (at least 24 weeks after the first dose).
2. The final dose in the series should be administered at least 6 months after the previous dose.
3. The minimum interval between the 2 doses of MMR vaccine is 4 weeks.
4. For persons aged 7 through 12 years, the recommended minimum interval between doses is 3 months. However, if the second dose was administered at least 4 weeks after the first dose, it can be accepted as valid. For persons aged 13 years and older, the minimum interval between doses is 4 weeks.

NCLEX-RN Flash Review

Part **V**

PEDIATRICS, DISORDERS

CHILD ABUSE: GENERAL

. . . .

CHILD ABUSE: TYPES

PART
V

. . . .

Definition: Purposeful maltreatment of a child.
Facts: Children less than 1 year old at highest risk for physical abuse; abuse often associated with a crisis or stressful event.
Assessment Findings: Varies according to type of abuse.
Nursing Interventions: Approach child slowly and at eye level; assess injuries and document findings; allow child to verbalize feelings/thoughts; reassure child that abuse is not his or her fault; report suspected abuse to proper authorities; if working with parents in follow-up care, assist in the identification of stressors and appropriate management and refer parents to appropriate community support systems.

. . . .

Type of Abuse	Symptoms
Physical	Unexplained injury or incongruous history of injury; bruises and fractures at varying levels of healing; bruises circling extremity; burns to extremities with specific shapes and patterns; hyperalertness when caregivers give directions; overeagerness to please; frightened by adults.
Shaken Baby Syndrome	Intercranial hemorrhage from vigorous shaking; swelling of head; bulging fontanels.
Neglect	Old dirty clothing; poor hygiene; lack of adult supervision; fatigue; poor school attendance; hunger.
Psychological	Poor self-esteem, acting-out behaviors, sucking, biting, rocking, poor academic performance, lack of friends and involvement in after-school activities, self-defeating/mutilating behaviors, suicide ideation.
Sexual	Bruises/bleeding in genital/anal area; changes in sleep pattern; poor self-esteem; sexually transmitted diseases; abnormal discharge/odor from genitals; enuresis.

. . . .

AORTIC STENOSIS

. . . .

ATRIAL SEPTAL DEFECT

PART
V

. . . .

COARCTATION OF AORTA

Definition: Narrowing of aortic valve that decreases blood flow from the left ventricle. This causes blood to be shunted from the left to the right side of the heart.

Causes: Progressive wear and tear of bicuspid valve present since birth (congenital); wear and tear of the aortic valve in elderly; scarring of aortic valve due to rheumatic fever as a child or young adult.

Assessment Findings: Congested cough, diaphoresis, fatigue, tachycardia, tachypnea.

Treatment: Surgery.

Nursing Interventions: Monitor vitals, pulse oximetry, intake and output; cardiac assessment for early signs of decomposition; daily weights; high-calorie diet with easy-to-digest food; keep head elevated (may place infant in car seat to do this).

Special Consideration: While infant is usually acyanotic, may present with mild cyanosis.

· ·

Definition: Birth defect resulting in an abnormal opening between the right and left atria of the heart.

Causes: Congenital birth defect.

Assessment Findings: Infant may be asymptomatic or may have difficulty feeding; exercise intolerance; oliguria; pale, cool extremities; tachycardia; periods of cyanosis; jugular vein distension; peripheral edema and/or symptoms of respiratory distress.

Treatment: Closure of the opening via cardiac catheterization or open repair with bypass surgery.

Nursing Interventions: Monitor vital signs; assess for signs and symptoms of congestive heart failure and/or decreased cardiac output; weigh daily; provide small, frequent feedings to conserve energy; administer oxygen, medication, and fluid restrictions as prescribed.

Special Consideration: Repair of defect is usually done before the child reaches school age.

· ·

Definition: Narrowing of the aorta near the ductus arteriosus.

Cause: Congenital birth defect.

Assessment Findings: Blood pressure is higher in the upper extremities than the lower extremities; bounding pulses in arms, cool lower extremities, weak/absent femoral pulses; headaches, nosebleeds, dizziness, signs of congestive heart failure or decreased cardiac output.

Nursing Interventions: Monitor blood pressure and pulses in all extremities; assess for decreased cardiac output, congestive heart failure; administer oxygen and medication as prescribed.

Treatment: Angioplasty with balloon; surgical management via resection and end-to-end anastomosis of constricted section.

Special Consideration: Cardiac bypass surgery is not usually necessary.

CONGESTIVE HEART FAILURE

· ·

HYPOPLASTIC LEFT-HEART SYNDROME

· ·

JONES CRITERIA

PART
V

Definition: The heart is unable to effectively pump the blood volume needed to meet the infant's/child's metabolic needs.
Cause: Usually caused by a congenital heart defect that then leads to congestive heart failure.
Assessment Findings: Tachypnea, tachycardia, cyanosis, difficult feeding, edema, diaphoresis, signs/symptoms of respiratory distress, ascites, jugular vein distension, oliguria, weight gain, poor growth.
Nursing Interventions: Monitor vital signs and respiratory status; elevate head of bed, maintain strict intake and output, decrease stimulation, small frequent feedings; administer oxygen, digoxin, diuretics, angiotension-converting enzyme inhibitors, sedatives as ordered.

. . . .

Definition: Underdevelopment of left side of heart.
Cause: Congenital birth defect.
Assessment Finding: Symptoms progress from mild cyanosis and symptoms of congestive heart failure to severe decrease in cardiac output and eventually cardiac collapse.
Treatment: Requires mechanical ventilation with administration of prostaglandin E1 to ensure adequate blood flow until surgical intervention is completed. Transplantation may be considered.
Special Consideration: Without intervention, hypoplastic left-heart syndrome is fatal.

. . . .

Definition: Used to diagnose rheumatic fever; consists of two categories: major criteria and minor criteria. *Major criteria* include carditis, painful joints, involuntary movements (chorea), erythema marginatum, and subcutaneous nodules. *Minor criteria* include fever, elevated sedimentation rate, positive c-reactive protein, and prolonged P-R interval. According to Jones criteria, the child must have evidence of preceding streptococcal infection of the throat plus exhibit two of the major symptoms or one major and two minor symptoms for a diagnosis of rheumatic fever to be made.

PATENT DUCTUS ARTERIOSUS

. . . .

PULMONARY ARTERY STENOSIS

. . . .

RHEUMATIC HEART DISEASE (RHD)/
RHEUMATIC FEVER (RF)

PART V

Definition: Abnormal opening between the aorta and pulmonary artery that causes blood from the aorta to be shunted to the pulmonary artery.
Causes: Congenital disorder where the ductus arteriosus fails to close after the birth.
Assessment Findings: Machinelike murmur; widened pulse pressure; bounding pulses; difficulty feeding; exercise intolerance; oliguria; pale; cool extremities; tachycardia; periods of cyanosis; jugular vein distension.
Nursing Interventions: Monitor vital signs; assess for signs and symptoms of congestive heart failure and/or decreased cardiac output; weigh daily; provide small frequent feedings to conserve energy; administer oxygen, medication, and fluid restrictions as prescribed.
Treatment: Medication (Indocin/Indomethacin), cardiac catheterization, or surgical intervention to close defect.
Special Consideration: Infant may be asymptomatic except for machine-like murmur.

. . . .

Definition: Narrowing of the pulmonary artery; leads to decreased pulmonary blood flow and right ventricular hypertrophy.
Cause: Congenital birth defect.
Assessment Findings: Heart murmur; exercise intolerance; oliguria; pale, cool extremities; tachycardia, periods of cyanosis, jugular vein distension, peripheral edema, and/or symptoms of respiratory distress; may also be asymptomatic.
Treatment: Dilation of constricted area via cardiac catheterization or surgical management.
Nursing Interventions: Monitor vital signs; assess for signs and symptoms of congestive heart failure and/or decreased cardiac output; weigh daily; provide small, frequent feedings to conserve energy; administer oxygen, medication, and fluid restrictions as prescribed.

. . . .

Definition: Inflammatory disease that can cause permanent damage to the heart valves with the mitral valve and aortic valve most commonly involved.
Causes: RHD is a complication of rheumatic fever; RF typically occurs 2 to 6 weeks after a partially treated or untreated streptococcal throat infection.
Assessment Findings: *RHD:* Shortness of breath, fatigue, chest pain, tachycardia, palpitations, prolonged P-R interval. *RF:* Joint pain, irregular, involuntary movements (chorea); fever, erythema marginatum (rash common in RF); elevated sedimentation rate and antistreptolysin O titer; subcutaneous nodules over joints.
Nursing Interventions: *RF:* Monitor vital signs; administer aspirin and antibiotic therapy as ordered; teach parents home medication management: s/s aspirin toxicity, need to complete antibiotic therapy, including monthly prophylactic antibiotic if ordered. *RHD:* Assess for decreased cardiac output and congestive heart failure; administer digoxin and diuretics as ordered.
Special Consideration: Child may need prophylactic antibiotic therapy for dental work, infections, and invasive therapies.

TETRALOGY OF FALLOT

. . . .

TRANSPOSITION OF GREAT VESSELS

PART V

. . . .

TRUNCUS ARTERIOSIS

Definition: Abnormality of the heart that involves four defects: ventral septal defect, pulmonary stenosis, overriding aorta (aorta is over and above ventral septal defect), and right ventricular hypertrophy.
Cause: Congenital birth defect.
Assessment Findings: "Tet" or "blue" spells: hypoxic episodes relieved by squatting or knee chest position; spells often occur during feeding and crying; cyanosis, murmur, clubbing of fingers, poor growth.
Treatment: Surgical management via palliative shunt or complete repair; palliative shunting is done to increase blood flow to pulmonary artery when child is unable to undergo repair.
Nursing Interventions: During "tet" or "blue" spells: calmly place child in knee chest position; administer 100% oxygen via face mask, morphine sulfate, IV fluids per physician order; document occurrence, preceding event, actions taken, and infant's response.

. . . .

Definition: Reversal of aorta with the pulmonary artery so that the aorta leaves the right ventricle and the pulmonary artery leaves the left ventricle.
Cause: Congenital heart defect.
Assessment Findings: Acutely cyanotic at birth due to lack of communication between systemic and pulmonary circulatory systems; if the child also has a ventral septic defect, patent ductus arteriosis or atrial septal defect cyanosis may be less severe.
Treatment: Administration of prostaglandin E to keep ductus arteriosis patent; atrial septostomy via cardiac catheterization to create an atrial septal defect until surgery can occur; surgical resection of aorta and pulmonary artery, then reattachment in correct anatomical positions to correct circulation.
Nursing Interventions: Administer medications per physician order and prepare infant for cardiac catheterization or surgery; provide emotional support to parents.
Special Consideration: Transposition of the great vessels is considered a medical emergency.

. . . .

Definition: Pulmonary artery, aorta, and coronary arteries form one arterial "trunk" and the aortic and pulmonary valves are combined into one truncal valve. A large ventral septal defect is also present.
Cause: Congenital heart disease stemming from failure of the aorta and pulmonary artery to divide during the embryonic period.
Assessment Findings: Loud continuous murmur; characteristic click from closing of truncal valve; mild cyanosis, signs and symptoms of congestive heart failure.
Treatment: Requires surgical correction, usually within the first months of life.
Nursing Interventions: Monitor vital signs; assess for cyanosis, signs/symptoms of congestive heart failure; administer oxygen and medications per physician order; provide emotional support to parents.

VENTRAL SEPTAL DEFECT (VSD)

. . . .

Definition: Abnormal opening between the right and left ventricles that causes blood to be shunted from the left ventricle to the right atrium. Can lead to left ventricle enlargement and pulmonary congestion.

Cause: Congenital heart defect.

Assessment Findings: Small VSD may be asymptomatic; loud murmur, tachypnia, diaphoresis, fatigue, underweight, tiring before feeding complete; symptoms of congestive heart failure.

Treatment: Small VSDs typically close without treatment; larger VSDs are treated with digoxin and diuretics until surgical repair occurs; surgery usually performed between 3 and 12 months of age; surgical closure may be completed via cardiac catheterization or bypass surgery.

Nursing Interventions: Monitor vital signs; assess for signs and symptoms of congestive heart failure and/or decreased cardiac output; weigh daily; provide small frequent feedings to conserve energy; administer oxygen, medication, and fluid restrictions as prescribed.

Special Consideration: Most common congenital heart disease.

. . . .

DEHYDRATION

....

DIABETES MELLITUS

....

FEVER

Definition: Loss of extracellular fluid leading to fluid and electrolyte imbalance.

Causes: Vomiting, diarrhea, burns, hemorrhage, adrenal insufficiency.

Assessment Findings: Weight loss, increased pulse, depressed or sunken anterior fontanel, decreased blood pressure, dry mucous membranes, decreased urinary output, decreased or absent tears.

Treatment: Treatment of underlying cause and correction of fluid and electrolyte imbalance; oral rehydration via Pedialyte, Infalyte, or similar product for mild to moderate dehydration; IV hydration and electrolyte replacement for severe dehydration.

Nursing Interventions: Assess vital signs, intake and output; monitor for signs of dehydration; administer fluid and electrolytes per order.

Special Considerations: Athletic drinks like Gatorade and Powerade should not be utilized due to their high carbohydrate and low electrolyte concentrations; fruit juices and carbonated beverages should also be avoided.

. . . .

Definitions: *Type 1:* Inability of the pancreas to produce insulin, causing altered ability to metabolize carbohydrates and lipids. *Type 2:* Inability of the body to utilize insulin effectively due to insulin resistance.

Causes: Combination of genetic, autoimmune, and environmental factors; obesity increases risk for type 2 diabetes.

Assessment Findings: Polydipsia (increased thirst), polyphagia (increased hunger), polyuria (increased urination); enuresis; weight loss, fatigue, nausea and vomiting, headaches, fruity-smelling breath.

Treatment: Blood glucose monitoring; diet and exercise counseling and management; augmentation of insulin production via medication (type 2); insulin administration via subcutaneous injections or pump (Type 1).

Nursing Interventions: Monitor glucose levels and administer insulin as ordered; teach child and caregivers home management of diabetes, including medication or insulin administration, monitoring and recording of glucose levels, nutrition and exercise guidelines, signs/symptoms and management of hypo-/hyperglycemia, sick day management.

Special Consideration: Type 2 diabetes is on the rise in children and adolescents.

. . . .

Definition: Elevation of body temperature to greater than 38°C or 100.4°F.

Causes: Viral or bacterial infection.

Assessment Findings: Elevated temperature, skin that is warm and/or flushed, diaphoresis, lethargy.

Nursing Interventions: Assess vital signs and for signs/symptoms of dehydration; administer cool compress to forehead, tepid sponge bath; administer acetaminophen or ibuprofen per order; avoid use of aspirin due to risk for Reye's syndrome.

Special Considerations: Temperatures in children fluctuate throughout the day and with activity and emotional distress. The axillary or tympanic route should be utilized to take the child's temperature until the child is >5 or 6 years of age.

PHENYLKETONURIA

Definition: Blood level of phenylalanine to greater than 20 mg/dl; toxic levels of phenylalanine lead to central nervous system damage.

Cause: Autorecessive genetic disorder.

Assessment Findings: Phenylalanine blood level greater than 20 mg/dl; seizures; frequent vomiting; failure to gain weight; musty odor of urine; irritability, hyperactivity.

Treatment: Restriction of phenylalanine intake.

Nursing Interventions: Monitor growth and development; teach parents to limit child's phenylalanine intake through special formulas and avoidance of meat and dairy products as well as products containing aspartame.

Special Considerations: Newborn screening is required by law. Screening is completed using the Guthrie test. If the test is completed prior to 48 hours after birth, it should be repeated before the child is 14 days of age.

. . . .

APPENDICITIS

· ·

CELIAC DISEASE

· ·

CLEFT LIP/PALATE

PART V

Definition: Inflammation of appendix (small sac at end of cecum).
Causes: Blockage of appendiceal lumen from feces, parasites, enlarged lymph tissue, trauma to abdomen.
Assessment Findings: Pain that starts in the periumbilical area and then moves to right lower quadrant of the abdomen; rebound tenderness (pain upon removal of hand during deep palpation); referred pain; anorexia; nausea, vomiting, and/or diarrhea; elevated white blood cell count; abdominal guarding, fever.
Treatment: Surgical removal of appendix.
Nursing Interventions: Monitor vital signs; assess for signs and symptoms of *peritonitis*: sudden relief of pain followed by increased pain, increased fever, progressive abdominal distension, pallor, chills, increased heart rate, and increased respirations.

. . . .

Definition: Accumulation of glutamine in the blood due to intolerance of gluten (protein component of wheat, barley, rye, and oats). This leads to damage of the small intestine's mucosa and subsequent malabsorption.
Cause: Genetic disorder.
Assessment Findings: Chronic diarrhea; clay-colored, foul-smelling, greasy stool due to large amounts of unabsorbed fat (steatorrhea); anorexia; weight loss; irritability; abdominal distension.
Treatment: Avoidance of gluten in the diet.
Nursing Interventions: Nutritional consultation for gluten-free diet; reinforce need to eliminate gluten from diet by eliminating wheat, barley, rye, and oats; allow parent/child to verbalize feelings relating to gluten-free diet, and provide emotional support.
Special Consideration: Second most common cause of malabsorption in children.

. . . .

Definition: Abnormal opening in the lip and/or palate; *Unilateral:* Cleft located on one side of lip and/or palate. *Bilateral:* A cleft is located on both sides of the lip and/or palate.
Cause: Congenital abnormality where the soft tissue or bony structure of the lip and/or palate fails to fuse during embryonic development.
Assessment Findings: Ranges from slight notch to complete separation of lip/palate.
Treatment: Surgical correction.
Nursing Interventions: Assess extent of cleft via visualization and palpation with gloved finger; assess infant's ability to suck, swallow, feed; keep infant in upright position for feedings and keep bulb syringe and suction equipment at bassinette/crib; allow parents to verbalize feelings, and provide emotional support; encourage parental bonding with infant.

ESOPHAGEAL ATRESIA/ TRACHEOESOPHAGEAL FISTULA

. . . .

HIRSCHSPRUNG'S DISEASE

PART
V

. . . .

INTESTINAL PARASITES: GIARDIASIS

Definition: A condition in which the esophagus does not fully develop, causing it to end before it reaches the stomach. *Esophageal fistula* is a fistula that develops between the trachea and esophagus. Esophageal atresia and esophageal fistula typically occur together.
Cause: Congenital abnormality.
Assessment Findings: Copious, frothy bubbles in mouth; coughing; choking; cyanosis; abdominal distension; increased respiratory distress during and after feedings.
Treatment: Surgical repair.
Nursing Interventions: Monitor vital signs and respiratory status; maintain NPO (nothing by mouth) status, suction mouth secretions as needed; administer oxygen and IV therapy, antibiotics, and parental nutrition as ordered; keep head elevated.
Special Consideration: High risk for aspiration pneumonia.

. . . .

Definition: Absence of the parasympathetic nerve ganglion cells in the large intestine, causing severe constipation and intestinal blockage; also known as *congenital aganglionic megacolon*.
Cause: Congenital disease.
Assessment Findings: *Newborns:* Not passing meconium stool; bloody diarrhea; vomiting dark green or brown emesis; abdominal swelling; gas; reluctance to breast-bottle-feed. *Toddlers/older children:* Foul-smelling stool, fever, lack of energy, anemia, retarded growth, gas, bloody diarrhea, abdominal swelling; inability to pass stools without use of laxatives/enemas; severe constipation.
Treatment: Surgery: temporary colostomy to allow for bowel rest followed by removal of aganglionic bowel section with anastomosis of normal bowel and reversal of temporary colostomy.
Nursing Interventions: Monitor for signs and symptoms of bowel obstruction; nursing measures to prepare child for surgery; teach caregivers ostomy management; encourage verbalization of feelings and provide emotional support.

. . . .

Definition: Intestinal parasite that causes gastrointestinal distress; prevalent in crowded environments.
Cause: Protozoa.
Assessment Findings: Abdominal cramps; constipation alternating with loose stools; anorexia; steatorrhea; vomiting.
Nursing Interventions: Educate caregivers and children on proper hand washing and sanitary practices; encourage compliance with prescribed medication regime (metronidazole, tinidazole, nitazoxanide, or albendazole).
Special Consideration: Can spontaneously resolve in 4 to 6 weeks.

INTESTINAL PARASITES: PINWORMS

. . . .

INTUSSUSCEPTIONS

. . . .

OMPHALOCELE

Definition: Intestinal parasite that causes gastrointestinal distress; present in temperate climates.

Causes: Swallowing eggs of pinworms; most often occurs when someone with pinworms scratches around anus, getting the eggs on his or her hands, and then touches a surface or handles food that is later touched or eaten by the child.

Assessment Findings: Perianal itching/scratching; restlessness; disturbed sleeping patterns; enuresis.

Nursing Interventions: Teach caregiver and child proper hand washing; encourage all family members to comply with prescribed medication regime (Vermox, Pin-Rid, Albenza).

Special Considerations: Pinworms can be visually detected via inspection of anus with flashlight after child is asleep for 2 to 3 hours; often diagnosed via tape test, which consists of placing loop of transparent tape in child's perianal area and removing it in the morning for analysis.

· ·

Definition: One part of the intestine is prolapsed into another, blocking passage of food or causing the prolapsed portion of the intestine to die.

Causes: Not known.

Assessment Findings: Sudden loud crying; colicky abdominal pain; drawing up of knees to chest; vomiting bile-stained emesis; bloody, mucous stools (currant jelly stools); hypo or hyper bowel sounds; distended abdomen; fever; shock.

Treatment: Hydrostatic reduction: pressure from air or fluid is used to release the prolapsed intestine; surgery.

Nursing Interventions: Assess vital signs; monitor for signs of shock; administer antibiotics and IV fluids as prescribed; insert nasogastric (NG) tube if ordered; monitor for return of normal bowel functioning posttreatment.

· ·

Definition: Congenital malformation where abdominal contents herniate outside of the abdomen, usually in the umbilical area; abdominal viscera are covered with a protective sac; it is caused by a failure of the intestines to reenter the abdominal cavity during the 7th week of gestation, and it is treated via surgery.

POISONING

....

POISONING: ASPIRIN/ACETAMINOPHEN/ CORROSIVES

....

Definition: Ingestion, inhalation, or exposure to substance that interferes with the body's normal functioning, causing harm to the body.

Causes: Most preadolescent episodes occur as accidents within the home.

Assessment Findings: Vary by poisoning agent.

Treatment: Varies by poisoning agent; may include: *Syrup of Ipecac:* Induces vomiting; use less common; contraindicated for corrosive substances. *Gastric lavage:* Used to empty the stomach within 1 to 2 hours of ingestion; contraindicated for corrosive substances. *Activated charcoal:* Decreases amount of toxic agent absorbed by GI system. *Cathartic agents:* Hasten expulsion of the substance by increased GI motility. *Antidotes:* Vary by type of poisoning.

Nursing Interventions: Monitor vital signs, airway, breathing, and circulation; administer oxygen; assist in identification of poison and administration of ordered treatment; educate all parents on modification of the home for child safety during infancy before the child can crawl.

Special Consideration: For toddlers and preschoolers, poisoning is the fourth leading cause of death and the leading cause of injury.

· ·

Poison	Symptoms	Treatment
Acetaminophen (Tylenol)	*General:* Nausea, vomiting, weakness, malaise, confusion, diaphoresis, drowsiness. *Hepatic:* Jaundice, right upper quadrant abdominal pain, stupor, increased liver and bilirubin levels. (*Note:* Hepatic symptoms may be irreversible.)	Administration of N-acetyl cysteine (Mucomyst); may be diluted in juice or soda to increase palatability.
Acetylsalicylic Acid (Aspirin)	Nausea, vomiting, tinnitus, hyperpnea, fever, confusion, sweating, seizures, oliguria, coma.	Activated charcoal; cathartics.
Corrosives	Burning in mouth, throat, stomach, vomiting, drooling.	Dilute corrosive with water or milk; do not induce vomiting.

· ·

POISONING: LEAD

. . . .

PYLORIC STENOSIS

. . . .

Definition: Accumulation of excessive levels or toxic levels of lead in the blood.

Causes: Commonly occurs through ingestion of lead-contaminated objects such as loose paint chips, pottery, or ceramic ware, or inhalation of lead dust within the environment.

Assessment Findings: Bone pain, constipation, increased intracranial pressure, changes in behavior or motor activity, weight loss, vomiting, peripheral neuritis, lead lines in gums.

Treatments: Chelation therapy; administration of calcium disodium edentate (EDTA).

Nursing Interventions: Assess vital signs; administer IV fluids, chelation therapy, medications as ordered; if EDTA prescribed, administer IM into large muscle mass to decrease pain; monitor calcium levels, intake and output, hydration and kidney functioning; teach parents preventive measures, medication administration, and need for continued follow-up.

Special Consideration: Screening occurs by assessment of blood levels of lead; guidelines vary by state but screening generally occurs between ages of 1 and 2 or earlier if in high-risk area.

· ·

Definition: Enlargement of the muscles surrounding the pylorus, causing a narrowing of the pyloric canal and blocking of food passage from stomach to intestines.

Cause: Progressive thickening of muscles surrounding pylorus.

Assessment Findings: Symptoms typically begin at 3 weeks of age and include vomiting that progresses from mild regurgitation to projectile; hunger after vomiting, decreased stools, constipation, mucous or bloody stools, dehydration symptoms, electrolyte imbalance.

Treatment: Pyloromyotomy: surgical procedure where muscles surrounding pylorus are cut to relieve constriction.

Nursing Interventions: Monitor vital signs, emesis, intake and output; assess for signs and symptoms of dehydration and electrolyte imbalances; assist in preparation of child and family for pyloromyotomy.

· ·

VOMITING/DIARRHEA

	Vomiting	Diarrhea
Causes	Increased intercranial pressure, virus, toxic ingestion, food intolerance, obstruction in GI tract.	Infectious diseases, antibiotic therapy, intestinal parasites, inflammatory bowel disease, food allergies, rotavirus.
Concerns	Aspiration, dehydration.	Dehydration.
Assessment	Characteristics of emesis s/s aspiration, dehydration, fluid and electrolyte imbalance.	Characteristics of stool, s/s dehydration, fluid and electrolyte imbalance.
Nursing Interventions	Maintain patent airway, monitor vital signs, emesis, force of vomiting, intake and output, s/s dehydration and electrolyte imbalance; provide oral rehydration.	Monitor vital signs, stool, intake and output, s/s dehydration and electrolyte imbalance, s/s dehydration; provide oral rehydration; provide IV hydration if ordered.

CRYPTORCHIDISM

. . . .

ENURESIS

. . . .

EPISPADIAS/HYPOSPADIAS

PART
V

Definition: Failure of one or both of the testes to descend into scrotal sac; usually self-resolves during first year of life; if not, surgery (orchiopexy) may be performed.

· ·

Definition: Child is unable to control bladder function even though child is of age to have bladder control or had control previously.
Causes: Delayed maturation of central nervous system, sleep disorders, urinary tract infections, other organic causes.
Assessment Findings: *Primary nocturnal enuresis:* Bed-wetting at night in child who has never been dry throughout night; child is unable to sense/awaken from full bladder.
Secondary/acquired enuresis: Occasional wetting after period of bladder control; may occur during night or day; dysuria, urgency, and/or frequency may also occur.
Nursing Interventions: Assist in assessment for underlying disease process such as urinary tract infection; encourage limited fluids at night, voiding prior to going to bed; encourage verbalization of child's and caregiver's feelings/concerns; provide emotional support; promote child's self-esteem.
Special Considerations: Bed-wetting is common in childhood; primary nocturnal enuresis usually self-resolves as the child matures.

· ·

Definition: Congenital defect where urethral opening of the penis is abnormally placed; circumcision is not usually performed, and surgical correction of the defect is usually conducted prior to the age of toilet training.
Epispadias: Opening is on dorsal side of penis.
Hypospadias: Opening is located on ventral side of the penis.

GLOMERULONEPHRITIS

. . . .

URINARY TRACT INFECTION

. . . .

PART
V

Definition: Kidney disorder where there is injury to glomerulus from inflammation.
Causes: Immunologic reaction; most likely antigen-antibody to group A streptococci elsewhere in the body.
Assessment Findings: Morning edema in face and periorbital area; urinary output that is decreased, cloudy, or bloody; proteinuria; lethargy; preceding infection or fever; elevated blood urea nitrogen (BUN) and serum creatinine; anorexia; fatigue; irritability; headaches.
Nursing Interventions: Assess vital signs, weight, intake, and urinary output; limit activities during acute phase; administer medications as ordered; diet restrictions of sodium and protein as ordered.

. . . .

Definition: Presence of microorganisms in the urinary tract causing infection.
Causes: Most common cause is *Escherichia coli*.
Assessment Findings: Vomiting, fever, poor feeding, failure to gain weight, diaper rash, enuresis, abdominal or back pain, blood in urine.
Nursing Interventions: Encourage fluids; teach prevention: wiping from front to back, especially in girls, changing stool-soaked diaper immediately; teach caregivers signs/symptoms of urinary tract infection and when to notify healthcare professional.

. . . .

CONJUNCTIVITIS (PINK EYE)

. . . .

OTITIS MEDIA

. . . .

PEDICULOSIS (LICE)

PART
V

Definition: Inflammation of the conjunctiva in the eye.
Causes: *Neonatal:* Chemical irritation or infection such as maternal chlamydia. *Childhood:* Allergy or bacterial/viral infection.
Assessment Findings: Itching, burning, red eyes; photophobia; discharge from eyes.
Nursing Interventions: Cold compresses to eye; reduced lighting; prevention of eye rubbing; administer prescribed eye ointments from inner to outer cannula; teach caregivers proper hand washing after touching child's eye; encourage use of separate towel, washcloth, and pillowcase for infected child.
Special Considerations: Child should not attend day care or school until infection is resolved or until 48 hours after treatment is initiated, depending on school district/state policy.

· ·

Definition: Inflammatory infection of the middle ear.
Causes: Bacteria.
Assessment Findings: Fever; pain; tugging at ears (dependent on child's age); otoscopic examination reveals red, bulging eardrum; enlarged lymph nodes.
Nursing Interventions: Teach home management: taking antibiotics as prescribed, including complete course of therapy; avoidance of bottle-feeding infant in a supine position to decrease risk for otitis media.
Special Considerations: To perform otoscopic exam on a young child, gently pull the pinna down and back.

· ·

Definition: Infestation of the head with *Pediculus humanus capitis*.
Spread: Head-to-head contact or contact with hat, comb, bedding, or other personal item from infected person.
Assessment Findings: Persistent itching of the scalp, mild fever, malaise, presence of louse or nits (oval-shaped eggs).
Treatment: Pediculocides (Nix, Kwell, Scabene) and removal of nits.
Nursing Interventions: Teach caregivers hair care: wash child's hair with regular shampoo, then apply pediculocide according to manufacturer's instructions; following application, wet hair should be combed with fine-tooth comb to remove all nits; work with small sections of the hair from the scalp outward; teach cleansing of all potentially contaminated items by washing in hot water >120°F, having items dry-cleaned, or placing them in sealed bag for two weeks; soak combs and brushes in rubbing alcohol or boiling water; vacuum floors and furniture.

ALLERGIES

· ·

HEMOPHILIA

· ·

PART V

Definition: Abnormal response of the body to a substance.

Cause: IgE antibodies react with the substance, releasing histamines and causing visible signs and symptoms of a reaction.

Assessment Findings: Nausea, vomiting, diarrhea, blood in stools, itchiness; hives; wheezing, coughing, sneezing, runny nose. *Anaphylactic:* Swelling of lips, mouth, throat; tightening of throat; difficulty breathing; wheezing; coughing.

Nursing Interventions: *Anaphylactic symptoms:* Administer epinephrine and diphenhydramine per order. *General:* Educate caretaker and child on avoidance of foods containing allergen and/or reduction of exposure to environmental allergens; teach anaphylactic signs and symptoms and management (include use of epipen if ordered); allow caretaker and child to verbalize feelings and fears related to allergy and provide support. *Prevention:* Encourage breast-feeding for the first 6 months; encourage avoidance of cow's milk, eggs, fish, and peanuts during first year.

Special Considerations: Common food allergens include milk, eggs, soy, wheat, tree nuts, fish, shellfish, peanuts; small amounts of allergen can be transmitted through breast milk and cause a reaction.

• •

Definition: A group of disorders in which a deficiency of specific coagulation proteins causes bleeding; common types include A (factor VIII deficiency) and B (Christmas disease, factor IX deficiency).

Causes: Genetic; X-linked recessive disorder; mutation of specific gene.

Assessment Findings: Excessive or abnormal bleeding; bleeding after circumcision; nosebleeds; joint swelling, pain, warmth, or tenderness; tendency to bruise easily; prolonged PTT.

Treatment: *A:* Frozen factor VIII (cryoprecipitate); desmopressin acetate (DDAVP). *B:* Concentrated factor IX.

Nursing Interventions: Monitor for s/s bleeding; institute bleeding precautions; administer replacement factors as ordered; elevate, ice, and immobilize impacted joints; encourage avoidance of contact sports, and the use of helmets, knee pads, and elbow pads for bike riding and skating; teach signs/symptoms of bleeding and management of same; teach home administration of factors if administration is to be done at home.

• •

LEUKEMIA

. . . .

SICKLE-CELL ANEMIA

. . . .

Definition: A cancer of the white blood cells in which production is increased, causing release of blast cells (immature blood cells) versus mature white blood cells into the blood.

Causes: Virus, chemical exposure, genetics, radiation (ionizing).

Assessment Findings: Blood in emesis, bloody stools, hematuria, bone/joint pain, fatigue, history of frequent infections; low-grade fever, swelling of lymph nodes, petechia, bruising, blue/purple circles under eyes; blast cells in blood stream, white blood cell count <10,000.

Treatment: Chemotherapy, radiation therapy, bone marrow transplant, transfusions.

Nursing Interventions: Monitor vital signs and intake/outputs; teach/encourage high-protein diet with no raw fruits or vegetables; encourage avoidance of people with infectious diseases; perform interventions appropriate for treatment being administered; encourage verbalization of caregivers' and child's feelings; offer emotional support.

• •

Definition: Disorder in which body makes sickle-shaped red blood cells that contain hemoglobin S versus hemoglobin A and have a decreased capacity to carry oxygen to the tissues.

Causes: Genetic; African Americans are at higher risk.

Assessment Findings: Fatigue, pallor, shortness of breath, dizziness, abdominal pain, joint pain, lethargy, irritability, fever, enlarged spleen, jaundice, decreased growth.

Vaso-occlusive crisis (clumping of cells in circulation): Hand-foot syndrome (tender, warm, and swollen hands and/or feet). *Sequestration crisis* (pooling of blood in the spleen): Enlarged spleen, jaundice. *Aplastic crisis:* Decreased production of red blood cells.

Nursing Interventions: Assess vital signs, hydration, oxygenation; administer pain medication, IV fluids as ordered; promote elevation of joints, do not elevate head of bed more than 30 degrees; encourage high-protein diet; encourage receipt of flu, pneumonia, and meningococcal vaccinations; teach prevention of activities that promote crisis, including high altitudes, excessive exercise, deep-sea diving, use of aspirin; encourage treatment at early signs of infectious disease/dehydration.

• •

ACNE VULGARIS (ACNE)

• •

DERMATITIS/DIAPER RASH

• •

ECZEMA

PART
V

Definition: Common skin disease of adolescence characterized by eruption of papules and/or pustules on face, chest, and/or back.
Causes: During teen years, sebaceous glands increase in size and production of sebum; the epithelial cells lining skin follicle become more cohesive and accumulate sebum and dead skin cells, effectively clogging the skin pore.
Assessment Findings: Papules and/or pustules on face, chest, back.
Nursing Interventions: Teach adolescent proper skin hygiene, avoidance of popping acne pimple, and correct administration of skin care treatment plan, including medications, topical creams, and cleansing agents.

• •

Definition: Macerations and lesions in the perineum.
Causes: Prolonged contact with urine or feces; reaction to foods.
Assessment Findings: Red, macerated skin with lesions.
Nursing Interventions: Assess for symptoms of candidiasis (yeast) infection such as beefy red erythemia with satellite lesions. Teach caregiver importance of changing diapers when soiled, cleansing thoroughly with wipe or gentle soap and water; application of barrier ointment or cream after skin is dried; exposure of affected skin to air several minutes each day.
Special Considerations: Candidiasis (yeast) infections require treatment with prescription antifungal cream/ointment.

• •

Definition: Inflammation of the epidermis.
Causes: Associated factors include family history of eczema, allergies, asthma.
Assessment Findings: Redness, scales, minute papules, lesions that weep, ooze, and/or crust; itchiness.
Nursing Interventions: Teach child and caregiver to avoid excessive bathing and exposure of skin to harsh soaps and detergents; encourage lubrication of skin after bathing; teach prescribed medication regime including antihistamines, topical corticosteroids, antibiotics (if infection occurs); encourage short, clean nails; teach signs/symptoms of skin infection and management of same.

IMPETIGO

PART V

Definition: Superficial bacterial skin infection.

Causes: Staphylococcus aureus or streptococcus pyogenes, methicillin-resistant staphylococcus aureus (MRSA).

Assessment Findings: Lesions, itchiness, burning, redness. *Nonbullous:* Small fluid-filled blisters that erupt and then form a tan or yellow/brown crust. *Bullous:* Large blisters filled with clear fluid that turns cloudy; blisters not as likely to erupt.

Nursing Interventions: Teach child and caregiver to allow lesions to air-dry, administer medications such as topical ointments and antibiotics as prescribed, use warm saline soaks to remove crusting, keep child's fingernails short and clean; use of separate towels and linens and proper hand washing technique.

NCLEX-RN Flash Review

BARLOW MANEUVER

· ·

HIP DYSPLASIA

· ·

JUVENILE RHEUMATOID ARTHRITIS

PART V

Definition: With infant lying supine, flex hips to 90 degrees. Place index and middle finger of greater trochanters and thumb at inner thigh inguinal crease. Gently adduct hip while applying gentle downward force. If a click is heard or felt, it is considered a positive response and is indicative of a hip dysplasia.

. . . .

Definition: Abnormal development of the hip during fetal period or childhood in which the femur is positioned incorrectly in the acetabulum; results in affected leg being shorter than nonaffected leg; treatment usually consists of open or closed hip reduction.

. . . .

Definition: Autoimmune disease causing inflammation of the joints.
Causes: Interaction of genetic, environmental, and immunological factors.
Assessment Findings: Stiffness and immobility of joints in the morning; joint pain; muscle pain; fatigue; malaise; lymphadanopathy; fevers; salmon-pink, migratory rash in late afternoon or evening; periods of exacerbation and remission of symptoms.
Treatment: Nonsteroidal anti-inflammatory drugs (NSAIDs), slow-acting anti-rheumatic drugs (SAARDs) such as sulfasalazine; methotrexate; corticosteroids.
Nursing Interventions: Assess range of motion and strength; apply heat or cold therapy; position joints to relieve pain and provide support; teach/ encourage adherence to prescribed medication regime, avoidance of contact sports and high-impact activities, alternating periods of activity with periods of rest.

MUSCULAR DYSTROPHY (DUCHENNE'S)

. . . .

ORTOLANTI'S MANEUVER

. . . .

SCOLIOSIS

PART
V

Definition: Disease that involves progressive muscular deterioration and generally results in death.
Causes: Genetic defect in the X chromosome that interferes with dystrophin production resulting in the breakdown of the muscle fibers.
Assessment Findings: Pelvic weakness, delayed motor development, waddling, walking on toes, marked lordosis, muscle weakness/wasting progressing from proximal to distal muscles. *Gowers' sign:* Having to use hands to push self up from squatting position.
Nursing Interventions: Encourage verbalization of feelings/fears; provide emotional support; assist child in maintaining self-esteem and reaching potential; offer parents genetic counseling; refer to physical therapy and appropriate community resources; teach caregivers prevention of respiratory infections and promote healthy diet and weight.
Special Consideration: There is no known cure for muscular dystrophy.

• •

Definition: Performed by flexing infant's hips and knees to 90 degrees. The healthcare provider then places index fingers on greater trochanters and applies gentle pressure while abducting infant's legs. If a click is heard or felt, it is considered a positive response and can be indicative of posterior dislocation of the hip.

• •

Definition: Lateral curvature of the spine accompanied by rotation of the vertebral column; may be structural (primary deformity) or functional (secondary to another problem); findings usually include unequal hip or shoulder heights, prominent scapula, curved spinal column, asymmetry of the back; treatment can involve electrical stimulation, bracing, or surgery.

ATTENTION-DEFICIT/ HYPERACTIVITY DISORDER (ADHD)

. . . .

AUTISM

. . . .

Definition: Learning disorder with characteristic inattention, hyperactivity, and/or impulsivity.

Causes: Unknown, but risk increases with first-degree relative with the disorder.

Assessment Findings: Inability to concentrate; easily distracted; appears to ignore instructions, tasks, or assigned chores; does not complete tasks; underachievement in school; excessive fidgeting; disruptive in classroom; interrupts others; impulsive.

Treatments: Pharmacotherapy and behavioral therapy.

Nursing Interventions: Educate caregivers on prescribed medication regime and home interventions: development of routines; clear, concise rules with appropriate consequences; assign one task at a time; break large tasks into smaller parts. Educate on schoolwork interventions: copies of schoolbooks at home; use of colored markers to highlight books; close communication with child's teachers. Allow child and caregiver to verbalize feelings/fears; provide emotional support; promote child's self-esteem.

. . . .

Definition: A developmental disorder that interferes with child's ability to communicate and interact with others.

Causes: Possibly genetic with environmental trigger; not caused by child-hood vaccinations.

Assessment Findings: Poor eye contact, failure to respond to name, poor communication skills, bizarre body movements, singsong voice, robotlike voice, sensitivity to tactile stimulation, altered response to pain, solitary play, behavior or play rituals, awkward gait, rocking, waving hands, banging head into objects.

Nursing Interventions: When caring for an autistic child, incorporate the caregivers in the planning of care; find out child's routines, likes and dislikes, response to pain, self-care needs; allow caregivers to verbalize feelings; provide emotional support.

. . . .

CEREBRAL PALSY

· ·

CEREBRAL PALSY: TYPES

· ·

PART
V

Definition: Nonprogressive neurological disorder that appears in infancy or early childhood and causes permanent motor dysfunction.

Causes: Abnormality in the section of the brain that controls motor movement, arising from congenital malformation or anoxia of the brain before/during/after birth.

Assessment Findings: Vary based on muscle responses: *Hypotonia:* Floppiness, diminished reflexes. *Hypertonia:* Rigidity, spasticity, scissoring of lower legs, exaggerated reflexes. *Athetosis:* Involuntary writhing motions. *Ataxia:* Uncoordinated muscle movement, wide-based gait.

Nursing Interventions: Assist in early recognition and implementation of early interventions to maximize child's potential; assess child's developmental level; encourage communication and interactions appropriate for child's developmental age; teach caregiver feeding methods to prevent aspiration, such as upright position and support of lower jaw; coordinate multidisciplinary care team, including physical therapist, occupational therapist, speech therapist, nutritionist, and orthopedics; allow family to verbalize feelings; offer emotional support; refer to appropriate community agencies/support groups.

Type	
Hemiplegia	Involves one side of body; upper extremities with greater dysfunction than lower.
Diplegia	Both sides of body involved; lower extremities with greater dysfunction than upper.
Quadriplegia	All four extremities involved equally.

HYDROCEPHALUS

. . . .

NEURAL TUBE DEFECTS

. . . .

PART
V

Definition: Increased retention of cerebral spinal fluid within ventricles of the brain.

Causes: Obstruction of blood flow between ventricles; increased risk with Dandy-Walker syndrome, spina bifida, meningitis.

Assessment Findings: *Infants:* Shrill cry, bulging fontanel, widening suture lines, sunset eyes. *Older children:* Change in level of consciousness, headache, vomiting, irritability, seizures, lethargy. *Both:* Decreased pulse, increased blood pressure.

Nursing Interventions: *Pre-op:* Elevate head of bed; prepare for surgical insertion of shunt from ventricle to peritoneum. *Post-op:* Assess for signs of shunt malfunction (signs of increased intercranial pressure); assess for signs of infection; teach client to watch for signs of increased intercranial pressure and to report immediately to physician, as shunt will need to be revised.

Special Consideration: Although shunt is designed to grow with child, the child will eventually outgrow shunt and need to have it replaced.

Ancephaly	Absence or decreased size of cerebral hemispheres; death usually occurs due to respiratory failure.
Cranioschisis	Protrusion of neural tissue through skull defect.
Exancephaly	Brain is totally exposed or protruding from skull defect.
Encephalocele	Saclike protrusion of brain and meninges through skull defect.
Spina Bifida	Posterior vertebral arch fails to fuse or fails to close.

REYE'S SYNDROME

. . . .

SPINA BIFIDA

. . . .

SPINA BIFIDA: TYPES/SYMPTOMS

PART
V

Definition: A disorder where cerebral edema and fatty changes in the liver occur after a viral illness; linked to use of aspirin in children; therefore, acetaminophen is the preferred medication; children and teenagers with flulike symptoms or chicken pox should never be given aspirin.

· ·

Definition: Birth defect of the central nervous system in which there is incomplete development of the spinal cord or its covering.
Causes: Failure of the neural tube to close during the first 28 days of gestation; folic acid deficiency has been linked to spina bifida.
Assessment Findings: Vary by type.
Nursing Interventions: Assess for hydrocephalus; measure head circumference daily; assess for signs of meningeal irritation such as fever and nuchal rigidity; if meningocele or myelomeningocele is present: position infant on abdomen, cover defect with normal saline dressing, prepare infant for surgery; allow parents to express feelings and fears; provide emotional support.

· ·

Type	Definition	Symptoms
Occulta	Failure of posterior vertebral arch to fuse without protrusions of the meninges.	Dimple or small depression noted at fifth lumbar vertebra or first sacral vertebra; may have abnormal gait and/or difficulty controlling bowel and bladder.
Cystica	Failure of posterior vertebral arch to fuse resulting in protrusion of the meninges.	*Meningocele:* Saclike herniation of the meninges and cerebral spinal fluid through a hole in the vertebrae; neurological deficits usually not present. *Myelomeningocele:* Saclike protrusion of meninges, cerebrospinal fluid, nerves, and a portion of the spinal column; neurological defects evident.

TRISOMY 21 (DOWN SYNDROME)

. . . .

Definition: Congenital disorder characterized by having an extra copy of chromosome 21; causes distinct physical attributes and decreased cognitive capabilities.

Cause: Incorrect/incomplete division/replication of chromosome 21.

Assessment Findings: Inner epicanthal eye folds, upper outer slant of eyes, flat and broad nose, protruding tongue, short neck, simian crease (palmar crease presenting as an unbroken line traveling straight across palmar surface), mental retardation; often accompanied by structural/functional cardiac and gastrointestinal disorders.

Nursing Interventions: Allow parents to verbalize feelings and offer emotional support; assess for feeding problems, cardiac and respiratory issues, delays in growth and development; refer to physical therapy, occupational therapy, speech therapy, and social services as needed.

Special Considerations: Trisomy 21 may be diagnosed during pregnancy via amniocentesis. Maternal serum alpha protein testing and fetal ultrasound may indicate Down syndrome during pregnancy but are not considered to be diagnostic tests.

ASTHMA

· ·

BRONCHOPULMONARY DYSPLASIA

PART V

· ·

CROUP (LARYNGOTRACHEOBRONCHITIS)

Definition: Reactive airway disease in which smooth muscles around the bronchi and bronchioles contract, causing a narrowing of the airway passages and/or causing the airways to become edematous and clogged.
Causes: Exposure to triggers such as allergens and cold air.
Assessment Findings: Tightness in the chest, cough, wheezing, retractions, decreased breath sounds, progressively worsening shortness of breath.
Nursing Interventions: Monitor respiratory status including pulse oximetry, respiratory effort, and lung sounds; administer oxygen, IV steroids, and nebulizer treatments per physician order; obtain blood gases per order; teach home management including identification/avoidance of asthma triggers, correct use of metered dose inhaler, and management of acute episodes, including when to seek emergency care.
Special Consideration: Parents should be taught to use fast-acting bronchodilators for symptomatic treatment.

• •

Definition: Chronic lung condition of newborns characterized by pulmonary changes such as bronchiolar metaplasia and interstitial fibrosis.
Causes: Risk factors include premature birth, long-term use of oxygen therapy, need for ventilator after birth.
Assessment Findings: Increased respiratory effort, nasal flaring, sterna retractions, increased respirations, elevated heart rate, crackles, rhonchi, wheezes, atelectasis.
Nursing Interventions: Monitor vital signs, assess cardiopulmonary status, provide oxygen or ventilator therapy as ordered; administer medications as ordered (surfactant, diuretics, corticosteroids, bronchodilators); teach parents home management, including oxygen therapy, tube feedings, and prevention of respiratory infections; allow caregivers to verbalize feelings/fears; offer emotional support.

• •

Definition: Swelling and inflammation of the upper airway leading to difficulty breathing and a "barking" cough.
Causes: Viral infection is the most common cause.
Assessment Findings: Barking cough, inspiratory stridor, elevated temperature; coldlike symptoms prior to onset.
Treatment: Most cases of mild croup are managed at home with cool mist humidifier therapy; moderate croup is managed through the emergency department with cool mist, aerosolized treatments, steroids; severe croup is treated with nebulized racemic epinephrine and/or hospitalization.
Nursing Interventions: Monitor vital signs, oxygen saturations; administer aerosolized treatments and medications as prescribed; provide cool mist or oxygen as ordered; assess hydration status and encourage intake of cool fluids.
Special Consideration: Symptoms are often worse at night.

CYSTIC FIBROSIS

· ·

EPIGLOTTITIS

· ·

**RESPIRATORY SYNCYTIAL VIRUS (RSV)/
BRONCHIOLITIS**

Definition: Chronic disease of lung and digestive system in which thick, viscous mucous is produced, causing clogging in the lungs and obstruction in the pancreas.
Cause: Genetic.
Assessment Findings: Salty-tasting skin; frequent respiratory infections; chronic productive cough; greasy, bulky, foul-smelling stools; wheezing, dyspnea; cyanosis; barrel chest; newborn meconium ileus; intestinal obstruction; delayed onset of puberty.
Nursing Interventions: Monitor vital signs, respiratory status, weight, signs of intestinal obstruction, blood glucose levels; encourage consistent administration of pancreatic enzyme replacements with meals and snacks; encourage deep-breathing exercises and chest physiotherapy or use of oscillating vest to loosen mucous; encourage adherence to high-protein, high-calorie diet with added salt; encourage verbalization of feelings/fears; provide emotional support; refer to appropriate community agencies.

• •

Definition: Life-threatening infection with inflammation and edema of the epiglottis.
Causes: Bacterial infection.
Assessment Findings: Extension of neck into a "sniffing" position, difficult and painful swallowing, increased drooling, restlessness, stridor, fever, cough, sore throat, tripod position when sitting.
Treatment: Emergency endotracheal intubation or tracheotomy.
Nursing Interventions: Monitor vital signs and oxygenation; decrease child's anxiety/stress; do not use tongue blade to inspect throat as this could cause epiglottis spasms and airway occlusion; prepare child/caregiver for endotracheal intubation or tracheotomy; allow caregiver to verbalize feelings/fears; offer emotional support.

• •

Definition: Bronchiolitis is a lung infection with production of thick mucus that causes occlusion and spasms of the bronchioles and small bronchi; the most common cause in children is RSV, a contagious disease spread by droplets of the virus sneezed or coughed into the air by an infected person.

SUDDEN INFANT DEATH SYNDROME (SIDS)

. . . .

SUDDEN INFANT DEATH SYNDROME (SIDS) RISK REDUCTION

. . . .

PART
V

Definition: Sudden, unexplained death of a healthy infant after being put to sleep.

Causes: Not known, but risk factors include low birth weight, history of siblings with syndrome, maternal smoking during pregnancy, sleeping in nonsafe sleep environment.

Assessment Finding: Death of the infant.

Nursing Interventions: Allow caregivers to verbalize feelings of loss, guilt, anger; provide emotional support; allow caregivers to cuddle infant and say good-bye; assist caregivers in contacting clergy if desired; refer to appropriate community agencies.

. . . .

Risk-reduction techniques include:
- Placing infant on back to sleep.
- Avoidance of bed sharing.
- Use of a crib with a firm mattress and a fitted sheet tight around mattress.
- Avoidance of pillows, blankets, stuffed animals, bumper pads in crib.
- Avoidance of soft surfaces for sleeping, such as couches, water beds, sofas, adult beds, toddler beds.
- Avoidance of smoking during pregnancy/after birth and near infant.
- Breast-feeding.
- Offering clean pacifier for sleep (if breast-feeding, offer pacifier after breast feeding firmly established).
- Dressing infant in light clothing and keeping room temperature at a comfortable level.

. . . .

Part **VI**

PEDIATRICS, MEDICATION

CALCULATIONS

. . . .

INTRAMUSCULAR INJECTIONS

PART
VI

. . . .

INTRAVENOUS BURETTE SETS

Pounds to Kilograms	Divide the child's weight in pounds by 2.2 (lbs/2.2 = weight in kilograms).
Kilograms to Pounds	Multiply child's weight in kilograms by 2.2 (kg x 2.2 = weight in pounds).
Milligrams per Kilogram per Day (mg/kg/day)	Milligrams to be administered multiplied by the child's weight in kg equals the total mg per day (mg x kg = milligrams per day).
Milligrams/Kilograms/Dose	Divide milligrams per day by number of doses to be given per day to get mg for each dose (milligrams per day/number of daily doses = mg per dose).

Developmental Stage	Needle Length	Preferred Location
Infant	$\frac{5}{8}$ inch	Vastis lateralis
Toddler	1 inch	Vastis lateralis Deltoid Rectus femoris
Preschooler	1 inch	Vastis lateralis Rectus femoris Ventral gluteal Dorsal gluteal Deltoid
Elementary School Age	1 to 1.5 inches	Vastis lateralis Ventral gluteal Dorsal gluteal Deltoid
Adolescent	1 to 1.5 inches	Vastis lateralis Rectus femoris Ventral gluteal Dorsal gluteal Deltoid

Definition: Microdrip set used for IV medication administration via piggyback to ensure exact delivery of small volumes of fluid; delivers 60 gtt/ml with a total capacity of 100 to 150 ml.

METERED DOSE INHALERS, ADMINISTRATION OF

. . . .

NASAL DROPS/OTIC DROPS, ADMINISTRATION OF

. . . .

ORAL MEDICATIONS, ADMINISTRATION OF

PART
VI

Administration technique:
- Have child exhale.
- As child is inhaling, administer medication.
- Have child hold breath 5 to 10 seconds.
- Have child exhale.

Use of spacer with metered dose inhaler:
- Have child exhale.
- Administer medication just prior to child inhaling.
- Have child inhale and hold breath for 5 to 10 seconds.
- Have child exhale.
- Have child inhale and hold breath 5 to 10 seconds.
- Have child exhale.

· ·

Nasal Medications	• Place child with head carefully hyperextended. (For younger child, have caregiver hold child on his or her lap with head extended over lap; have caregiver restrain child as needed.) • Administer nose drop, being careful not to let dropper touch nare. • Have child remain with head hyperextended for one minute.
Otic Medications	• Have child lie on side with affected ear exposed. (Younger child may be placed on caregiver's lap; have caregiver restrain child as needed.) • Gently pull pinna down and backward (young child) or up and outward (older child). • Administer medication. • Have child remain on side for one minute.

· ·

Techniques for administration:
- Mix suspensions thoroughly before pouring.
- Use firm, matter-of-fact approach.
- Use oral plastic syringe or measured medicine spoon, dropper, medicine cup, or nipple without the bottle attached, depending on child's developmental age.
- When using a dropper or oral syringe, direct liquid to the back and side of mouth, give in small quantities, and allow child to swallow.
- Small child may be placed across lap with child's dominant arm under adult's arm; child's head should be cradled in nondominant arm; administer medication slowly, directing liquid to the back and side of mouth.
- When using nipple without bottle, be careful to keep nipple full of medication to prevent air being taken in.

SUBCUTANEOUS INJECTIONS

Location	Center third of lateral aspect of upper arm. Abdomen. Center third of anterior thigh.
Procedural Tip	Pinch subcutaneous tissue to prevent injection into muscle.

Part **VII**

MENTAL HEALTH

ANXIETY

....

ANXIETY: GENERALIZED

....

Terms

Anticipatory Anxiety	Worry or fear about what will happen next.
Anxiety Trait	Responding to nonstressful situations with anxiety over a long period of time.
Anxiety State	Client loses control of his or her emotions in response to a stressful situation.
Free-Floating Anxiety	Worry or fear that is always present and may be accompanied by a feeling of dread.

Types of Anxiety

Mild	Worry or fear that is a part of living; it is perceived to be normal and can even produce positive outcomes by motivating or creating growth in an individual.
Moderate	Individual focuses on immediate concern and is selectively inattentive to other concerns.
Severe	Belief that something bad is going to happen; unable to focus on anything else.
Panic	Dread, terror, and/or sense of impending doom; perception becomes distorted; rational thought is lost.

. . . .

Definition: Unrealistic worry or excessive worry that occurs majority of the time; manifests with physical symptoms and is not caused by substance abuse and/or another medical condition
Cause: Multiple theories, including: (1) anxiety is a learned response, (2) stems from cultural factors, (3) genetic component, (4) biological component.
Assessment Findings: Varies by level of anxiety but includes elevated blood pressure and pulse; diaphoresis; hyperventilation; anorexia; sleep disturbances; dizziness; fatigue; inability to concentrate; pacing; nervous habits; decreased productivity; forgetfulness; inability to concentrate; withdrawal.
Treatments: Interventions are based on level of anxiety and include medication, cognitive-behavioral therapy, individual psychotherapy, and complementary therapies such as guided imagery, massage, and meditation.
Nursing Interventions: Utilize a nonjudgmental approach; assist client in meeting basic needs if needed; provide calm, nonstimulating environment; allow client to verbalize feelings; administer medications as ordered.

. . . .

OBSESSIVE-COMPULSIVE DISORDER

. . . .

PANIC DISORDER

. . . .

PART
VII

[455]

Definition: Recurrent, unwanted thoughts and fears that lead to repetitive behavior.

Causes: Theories include changes in body chemistry/brain function such as insufficient serotonin and behavior-related habits that were learned over time.

Assessment Findings: *Obsessions:* Involuntary, unwanted, repeated thoughts or images. *Compulsions:* Repetitive behaviors; often centers on themes such as cleanliness.

Treatment: Antidepressant medications; cognitive therapy.

Nursing Interventions: Use calm, nonjudgmental approach; provide safe environment for client to perform compulsive activity but encourage client to decrease amount of time engaged in activity; assist client in finding the meaning/reason for compulsive activity; assist client in identifying fear, and allow client to verbalize feelings; administer medications as ordered.

. . . .

Definition: Repeated attacks of intense fear or dread accompanied by physical symptoms that develop suddenly without warning, and intensify within ten minutes of onset.

Causes: Appears to have a genetic component and tends to occur during periods of life transitions.

Assessment Findings: Palpitations, chest pain, diaphoresis, dizziness, chills, hot flashes, tachycardia, shortness of breath, tingling or numbness in hands and feet, nausea, fear of impending doom.

Treatments: Medication; individual and group therapy.

Nursing Interventions: Utilize a nonjudgmental approach; assist client in meeting basic needs if needed; provide calm, nonstimulating environment; allow client to verbalize feelings; distract client from symptoms of panic attack; administer medications as ordered.

Special Consideration: Underlying medical conditions such as mitral valve prolapse, hypoglycemia, hyperthyroidism, and use of stimulants need to be ruled out.

. . . .

PHOBIA

. . . .

POST-TRAUMATIC STRESS DISORDER

. . . .

PART VII

Definition: Intense, irrational fear that results in avoidance of an object, activity, or situation.

Causes: Multifactor, including genetics, biological component, and/or precipitating traumatic event.

Assessment Findings: Symptoms occur when confronted with feared object/activity/situation and include intense fear or dread, desire to get away, chest pain, palpitations, shortness of breath, tremors, feeling of impending doom, tingling or numbness in hands and feet.

Nursing Interventions: Use calm, nonjudgmental approach; provide nonstimulating environment; assist client in identifying fear; allow client to verbalize feelings; administer medications as ordered.

· ·

Definition: Severe anxiety after experiencing, seeing, or learning about a traumatic event.

Cause: Traumatic event; it is not known why some people exposed to a traumatic event develop post-traumatic stress disorder and others do not.

Assessment Findings: Flashbacks, reliving experience and/or nightmares relating to experience; anxiety; attempts to avoid thinking/talking about event; emotional numbness; anger; irritability; sleep disturbances; hyperawareness; difficulty concentrating; difficulty maintaining close relationships.

Treatment: Anti-anxiety and antipsychotic medication, cognitive therapy.

Nursing Interventions: Use calm, nonjudgmental approach; allow client to verbalize feelings/details of the event; assist client in looking at event objectively; administer anti-anxiety and antipsychotic medications as ordered.

· ·

ALZHEIMER'S DISEASE

. . . .

AMNESTIC DISORDERS

. . . .

DELIRIUM

PART
VII

Definition: Physical changes in the brain leading to gradual loss of mental abilities, including executive functioning and memory impairment; progresses to disturbances in language, mood, personality, and motor functionality.

Causes: Combination of genetic, lifestyle, and environmental factors that lead to plaques (beta amyloid protein bundles that interrupt brain cells' ability to communicate) and tangles (twists of tau protein that inhibit transportation of key nutrients to brain cells), which lead to brain cell death and characteristic shrinkage of the brain.

Assessment Findings: Mild confusion, inability to organize thoughts, repetition of question/statements, forgetting family member names, misplacing items, becoming lost in familiar places, anger, irritability, and depression; disturbances in swallowing, bowel/bladder control, and muscle functioning.

Nursing Interventions: Approach client in a manner that allows client to retain dignity; keep communication clear and concise; allow client and caretaker to verbalize feelings; orient client to environment as needed; assist in management of activities of daily living as needed; administer medications as prescribed; consult social services as needed.

• •

Definition: Disorders that involve loss of previous memories, inability to create new memories, and loss of ability to learn new information.

Causes: May be caused by a medical condition, exposure to environmental toxin, or substance abuse.

Assessment Findings: Lack of orientation, confusion, inability to learn new information or create new memories; loss of memory of recent events.

Nursing Interventions: Provide safe environment, communicate with clear and concise statements, and allow for verbalization of feelings.

• •

Definition: Reversible state of attention and cognitive deficits precipitated by a definable event/cause.

Causes: Substance abuse, substance withdrawal, metabolic imbalances, infectious diseases, dementia.

Assessment Findings: Apathy, withdrawal, agitation, abnormal behavior that worsens at night, disorganized thinking, sleep disturbances, incoherent speech.

Nursing Interventions: Ensure safe, nonstimulating environment, assess degree of cognition impairment, institute measures to help client relax, administer medications per order.

Special Consideration: Treatment should begin with correction of underlying pathology.

VASCULAR DEMENTIA

. . . .

Definitions: Irreversible damage to brain tissue that leads to impairment in cognition, memory, and personality.

Causes: Narrowed blood vessels in brain from conditions such as diabetes, high blood pressure, and/or cerebral vascular incident.

Assessment Findings: Confusion, difficulty concentrating, memory loss, labile emotions, weakness, unsteady gait, wandering at night, decreased ability to organize thoughts.

Nursing Interventions: Provide calm, safe environment; allow client and caretaker to verbalize feelings; assist patient with lifestyle choices, including diet and exercise; assist client in managing underlying disease.

DELUSIONAL DISORDERS, GENERAL

....

DELUSIONAL DISORDERS, TYPES OF

....

Definition: Disorders characterized by fixed, lifelike, false beliefs not generally accepted by those in the client's culture.

Causes: Risk factors include low self-esteem, isolation, sensory deficits, severe stress, immigration, issues with trust and fear.

Assessment Findings: Delusions, hallucinations consistent with delusions; findings vary by type of delusional disorder.

Nursing Interventions: Establish trusting therapeutic relationship; set client goals; explore events triggering delusions; avoid arguing the reality of the delusion with client; administer medication as prescribed.

Delusional Disorder Subtype	Key Characteristics
Conjugal (Jealousy)	Belief that significant other is unfaithful.
Erotomania	Believes the existence of spiritual/emotional love from a person with an elevated social status.
Grandiose (Megalomania)	Client believes he or she has an unrecognized talent or insight.
Persecutory	Client believes there is a conspiracy against him or her.
Somatic	Belief that body parts are disfigured/nonfunctioning.

DEPERSONALIZATION DISORDER

. . . .

DISSOCIATIVE AMNESIA

. . . .

DISSOCIATIVE IDENTITY DISORDER

PART VII

Definition: Loss of one's personal reality via repeated or persistent feelings that things are not real; dreamlike state; feeling that one is observing oneself from outside the body.
Cause: Might be linked to imbalance of neurotransmitters; may be triggered by life-threatening event, fatigue, meditation, hypnosis, anxiety, severe pain; may also have no apparent trigger.
Assessment Findings: Feeling of detachment from body or mind; perceive self outside of body; feeling numb or robotic; impaired social functioning.
Nursing Interventions: Assist client to identify depersonalization as a coping mechanism; provide support; assist client in developing supportive relationships; teach effective self-management skills.

• •

Definition: Blocking out of certain information leading to loss of recall of personal information, memories, and/or traumatic event.
Causes: May have a genetic link; usually triggered by a traumatic event.
Assessment Findings: Sudden onset of inability to remember personal information, memories, and/or traumatic event.
Nursing Interventions: Encourage verbalization of feelings of distress; assist client in recognizing that memory loss is a defense mechanism; provide support; encourage development of supportive relationships and healthy coping mechanisms.
Special Consideration: Memories still exist but client has blocked their recall.

• •

Definition: Client has at least two distinct identities that control his of her behavior; different identities may have different physical characteristics, mannerisms, speech patterns, and/or gender identities.
Causes: Physical or sexual abuse; traumatic event occurring when the client was younger than age 15.
Assessment Findings: Presence of two or more distinct personalities; inability to remember events from a preceding time period; finding oneself somewhere and not knowing how one got there; people consistently knowing client that the client does not remember meeting; purchases that client does not remember buying; guilt; shame; low self-esteem; hallucinations; depression; self-mutilation; suicidal thoughts; substance abuse.
Nursing Interventions: Establish trusting therapeutic relationship; assess risk for self-harm and/or suicide and implement precautions as needed; encourage verbalization of feelings and of painful past experiences; explore coping mechanisms; focus on client's strengths; assist client in recognizing each personality and working toward integration; assist in identification of emotional responses to stress and development of healthy responses.

ANOREXIA NERVOSA

BULIMIA NERVOSA

Definition: Deliberate starvation or purging of self and a refusal/inability to maintain normal body weight.

Causes: Multifactor; risks include adolescence, low self-esteem, "model child" syndrome, sexual abuse, genetics, distorted body image.

Assessment Findings: Body weight less than 85% of normal weight for age/height; intense fear of gaining weight; preoccupation with thoughts of food; amenorrhea; depression; withdrawal from activities; insomnia; dry/flaky skin; constipation; decreased pulse and blood pressure; arrhythmias; lack of concern about symptoms.

Nursing Interventions: Establish trusting relationship; contract for amount of food to be eaten and/or weight to be gained; provide one-on-one support; encourage verbalization of feelings and perceptions of appearance; assist in identification/development of healthy coping mechanisms.

Special Considerations: Third most common chronic illness in adolescents; highest incidence involves high-achieving teenage girls; if left untreated, can be fatal; prevalence increasing in adult women.

. . . .

Definition: *Purging type:* Episodic periods of rapid consumption of large amounts of food in less than two hours followed by purging through induced vomiting and laxative abuse. *Nonpurging type:* Episodic periods of fasting and excessive exercise.

Causes: Common traits include viewing self as unlovable, inadequate, and/or unworthy; strong desire to please others; strong desire to be perfect, thin, loved, and/or accepted.

Assessment Findings: Binge eating, self-induced vomiting, abuse of laxatives, low self-esteem, mood disturbances, self-perception determined by body shape and weight, eroded tooth enamel, irregular/absent menses, arrhythmias. *Russell's sign:* Bruised knuckles from inducing vomiting.

Nursing Interventions: Establish trusting relationship; contract for amount of food to be eaten; prevent client from using bathroom within two hours of eating to prevent purging; provide one-on-one support; encourage verbalization of feelings and perceptions of appearance; assist in identification/development of healthy coping mechanisms.

. . . .

BIPOLAR DISORDER

. . . .

DEPRESSION

. . . .

Definition: Disruptive condition where client experiences periods of depression followed by periods of euphoria.

Causes: Increased risk associated with immediate family member with bipolar disorder, drug and alcohol abuse, periods of high stress.

Assessment Findings: *Manic phase:* Euphoria, decreased sleep, racing thoughts, impulsive actions, agitation, risky behavior, rapid speech, increased energy, lack of inhibition, spending sprees, increased sex drive. *Depressive phase:* Feelings of helplessness, hopelessness, suicidal thoughts, decreased alertness, sleep disturbances, poor hygiene, difficulty in thinking clearly, lack of interest in sex, apathy, increased absences from work or school.

Nursing Interventions: Approach clients with acceptance, honesty, empathy, patience and consistency; provide for physical needs such as rest, activity, nutrition as needed; assess suicide risk and implement suicide precautions if needed.

. . . .

Definition: Persistent feelings of sadness that interfere with the ability to eat, sleep, and enjoy activities that were once enjoyed.

Causes: Associated with biological, genetic factors, hormones, life events, and early childhood trauma.

Assessment Findings: *Mild:* Feelings of sadness that interfere with ability to engage in normal activities. *Moderate:* Feelings of helplessness, low energy levels, sleep disturbances, changes in appetite, weight; decreased concentration. *Severe:* Feelings of hopelessness, helplessness, and worthlessness; flat affect; changes in appetite/weight; sleep disturbances; constipation; loss of interest in sex; fatigue; inability to concentrate.

Nursing Interventions: Offer support by being with client; assess for level of depression; assess sleep, elimination, nutrition, and risk for suicide; implement suicide precautions if needed; use nondemanding approach to client interactions; allow client to verbalize feelings; initiate/implement safety contract with client; administer medications per order.

Special Considerations: Depressed clients are at increased risk for suicide; suspect thoughts of suicide if depressed client suddenly has improved mood or elation.

. . . .

SUICIDE

Definition: Taking of one's own life.

Causes: Risk increased by depression, previous suicide attempt, alcohol abuse, psychosis, drug abuse, individuals with lack of social support and/or a chronic illness.

Assessment Findings: The majority of potential victims give a clue before taking their lives, including talking about death, wanting to be dead, giving away cherished possessions, verbalizing feelings of helplessness and hopelessness, or saying that they want to harm themselves.

Nursing Interventions: Assess risk by asking clients if they have ever thought of harming themselves/taking their lives; if yes, ask if they have a plan for how they will take their lives; if client deemed at risk, implement suicide precautions (which may vary by organization but generally consist of someone staying with client at all times and removal of objects with which client could harm themselves).

Special Consideration: The more concrete the plan and the more available the tools for carrying out the plan, the more likely the client will attempt suicide.

ANTISOCIAL PERSONALITY DISORDER

....

BORDERLINE PERSONALITY DISORDER

....

DEPENDENT PERSONALITY DISORDER

Definition: Disorder in which client has total disregard for others' rights and has a track record of manipulating, exploiting, or violating others.
Causes: Believed to be linked to genetic factors and/or history of abuse as a child.
Assessment Findings: Destructive tendencies toward self and others; lack of remorse; manipulative behavior; ability to act witty and charming when desiring to do so; substance abuse; impulsiveness; history of breaking the law; inability to maintain personal relationships.
Nursing Interventions: Assess risk for self-harm/harm to others; provide safe environment; establish environment where client—but not maladaptive behavior—is accepted; encourage client to verbalize feelings; assist client identification of choices/actions that have caused difficulties; assist client in exploration of alternate coping mechanisms.

. . . .

Definition: Impulsive, unpredictable behavior that leads to unstable mood swings, interpersonal relationships, self-identity, and cognition.
Causes: Unknown but seem to be a combination of environmental and neurobiological factors.
Assessment Findings: Impulsive behavior relating to gambling, shopping, sex, and substance abuse; intense emotions; inability to maintain relationships; moodiness, low self-esteem, dysfunctional lifestyle; destructive behavior; frantic effort to avoid abandonment.
Nursing Interventions: Assess risk for self-harm/harm to others; provide safe environment; establish environment where client—but not maladaptive behavior—is accepted; encourage client to verbalize feelings; avoid reinforcement of manipulative behaviors; assist client in exploration of alternate coping mechanisms.

. . . .

Definition: Chronic disorder in which client relies too much on others to meet emotional and physical needs.
Causes: Not known.
Assessment Findings: Difficulty making everyday decisions; clinging, demanding behavior; difficulty expressing disagreement; going to excessive lengths to obtain nurturing from others; fear of losing people on whom the client depends.
Nursing Interventions: Establish trusting relationship; allow client to verbalize fears; assist client to make increasingly larger decisions and assume responsibility for self; help client identify manipulative behaviors; assist client in finding alternate coping mechanisms.

PARANOID PERSONALITY DISORDER

. . . .

Definition: Disorder that involves having an unwarranted and unrelenting mistrust and suspicion of others.

Causes: Not known.

Assessment Findings: Suspiciousness and mistrust of others; emotional distance; feelings of being deceived; disturbed sense of reality; low self-esteem; isolation; viewed as hostile, stubborn, and argumentative; reacts poorly to criticism.

Nursing Interventions: Establish therapeutic relationship; help client to identify negative behaviors that interfere with relationships; encourage socialization; assist in identification of positive behaviors and social skills.

. . . .

SCHIZOPHRENIA DISORDERS, OVERVIEW/ GENERAL PRINCIPLES

· ·

CATATONIC SCHIZOPHRENIA

· ·

DISORGANIZED SCHIZOPHRENIA

Definition: A group of disorders involving loss of reality and marked disturbances in thought, perception, and/or behavior.
Causes: Unknown combination of genetic, environmental, and biological
factors.
Assessment Findings: *Positive (distortion of normal functions):* Delusions
of persecution or grandeur, agitation, aggressive behavior, bizarre dress
or behavior, hallucinations. *Negative (decrease in normal functions):* Lack
of energy, withdrawal, difficulty thinking abstractly, lack of spontaneity, flat
affect, lack of self-initiated behaviors. *Disorganized:* Cognitive deficits,
disorganized/incoherent speech, repetitive rhythmic gestures.
Nursing Interventions: Establish trusting relationship, provide safe environment; offer clear, consistent, concise communications; assist client in
meeting basic physical needs; administer medication as ordered.

. . . .

Symptoms	Psychomotor disturbances. *Echolalia:* Repetition of a word or phrase. *Echopraxia:* Imitation of another's movements.
Nursing Interventions	Use touch judiciously.
Terms	*Catatonic stupor:* Vegetative-like condition. *Catatonic excitement:* Excessive motor activity.

. . . .

Symptoms	Personality disintegration; withdrawal; lack of attention to personal hygiene; hallucinations (sensory experiences that occur without external stimuli).
Nursing Interventions	Do not challenge client with hallucinations with reason. Do encourage clients with auditory hallucinations to verbalize what the voices are telling them to do.

PARANOID SCHIZOPHRENIA

. . . .

Symptoms	Delusions; auditory hallucinations; violent behavior.
Nursing Interventions	Set acceptable behavior limits. Provide calm, nonstimulating environment.

• •

GENDER DYSPHORIA

. . . .

PARAPHILIAS

. . . .

SEXUAL DYSFUNCTION

Definition: Disorder in which there is strong self-identification or desire to be a member of the opposite sex; strong discomfort with assigned gender.
Causes: Theories include genetic abnormality; hormone imbalance during fetal and childhood development; bonding deficits experienced in childhood.
Assessment Findings: Expressed desire to be/live as member of opposite sex; disgust with genitals; self-loathing/hatred; dressing as member of opposite sex; preoccupation with appearance; suicidal ideation; isolation, depression, and anxiety.
Treatments: Hormonal therapy, sex-reassignment surgery, group and individual therapy.
Nursing Interventions: Establish therapeutic relationship through caring, nonjudgmental approach; allow patient to verbalize feelings and fears; provide support; assist in client identification of strengths and positive aspects of self; assess risk for suicide, and implement precautions as appropriate.

• •

Definition: Sexual disorder where unusual sexual imagery or acts are utilized to achieve sexual excitement; involves nonhuman subjects, suffering/humiliation of oneself or partner, children, and/or nonconsenting adults.
Causes: Not known.
Assessment Findings: Utilization of nonhuman subject, child, nonconsenting adult, and/or suffering/humiliation to achieve sexual excitement; guilt and shame; disturbances in body image; sexual dysfunction; lifestyle changes to make object/method of excitement more accessible; emotional immaturity; need to prove masculinity (exhibitionists); poor self-concept; fear of sexual relationship that could cause rejection.
Treatment: Behavior, cognitive, and individual therapy.
Nursing Interventions: Utilize nonjudgmental approach; encourage client to identify feelings associated with sexual behavior/imagery.

• •

Definition: A sexual disorder presenting as a disturbance in one or more phases of the sexual response system and/or the presence of pain during intercourse not related to a physical cause.
Causes: Contributing factors include drugs/alcohol use, endocrine disorders, trauma, surgery, infections, medications, and pregnancy.
Assessment Findings: Varies by type of sexual dysfunction but includes decreased sexual desire, inability to become aroused, inability to maintain erections (in men), painful intercourse, poor self-concept, social isolation, anxiety, and fear of rejection.
Treatment: Varies with type of sexual dysfunction but includes medication adjustments, surgical implants, treatment of underlying medical conditions, vaginal dilators, and couples therapy.
Nursing Interventions: Provide safe, nonjudgmental relationship; encourage verbalization of feelings; discuss/teach alternate way of achieving sexual intimacy.

SEXUAL DYSFUNCTION, TYPES OF

Sexual Dysfunction Disorder	Definition
Sexual Desire Disorders	*Hypoactive:* Lack of sexual desire, causing distress to client or client's partner. *Aversion*: When confronted with sexual opportunity, client experiences fear, disgust, anxiety.
Sexual Arousal Disorders	*Females:* Little or no feelings of arousal. *Male:* Inability to obtain or maintain adequate erection (male erectile disorder, also known as erectile dysfunction).
Orgasmic Disorders	Recurrent episodes of inhibited orgasm after adequate period of arousal/excitement; category includes premature, inhibited, retarded ejaculation.
Sexual Pain Disorders	*Dyspareunia:* Recurrent genital pain during/after intercourse. *Vaginismus:* Vaginal spasms that interfere with sexual intercourse.

SOMATOFORM DISORDERS, OVERVIEW/ GENERAL PRINCIPLES

. . . .

BODY DYSMORPHIC DISORDER

. . . .

CONVERSION DISORDER

PART VII

Definition: A group of disorders that manifest as involuntary physiological symptoms that have no organic basis. Clients experience loss of function that significantly disrupts daily life and causes emotional distress.
Causes: Believed to have both biological and genetic factors.
Assessment Findings: Involuntary physical symptoms without organic basis; impairment in occupational, social, or other daily functioning; increased preoccupation with health including demand for unnecessary tests; failure to comply with treatment plans; traveling from healthcare provider to healthcare provider; excessive use of analgesics.
Nursing Interventions: Establish a trusting, nonjudgmental therapeutic relationship; encourage verbalization of feelings; assist client in moving focus from symptoms; assist client in identification of psychosocial needs being met by feeling unwell; assist in the development of alternate coping mechanisms.
Special Considerations: Although no organic reason exists for the client's physical symptoms, the symptoms are real to the client and cause significant distress and therefore should not be simply dismissed.

. . . .

Definition: A type of somatoform disorder in which there is a pervasive feeling of ugliness due to imagined or greatly exaggerated physical defect; negatively impacts client's social, occupational, or life functioning; also referred to as "imagined ugliness."

. . . .

Definition: A type of somatoform disorder with motor/sensory symptoms that are suggestive of a neurological condition, as anxiety is unconsciously converted into functional deficits.
Terms: *La belle indifference:* Client shows lack of appropriate concern for symptoms and does not manifest symptoms of anxiety (the symptoms of anxiety are transformed into symptoms that mimic physical ailments).
Pseudoneurological manifestation: Symptoms are present and resolve based on presence of life stress trigger.

HYPOCHONDRIA

. . . .

PAIN DISORDER

. . . .

SOMATIZATION DISORDER

PART
VII

Definition: A type of somatoform disorder in which physical complaints are exaggerated to the point that client experiences impairment in social or occupational functioning. Clients with this type of somatoform disorder typically travel from one healthcare provider to the next, as they feel that they are not receiving appropriate medical attention.

· ·

Definition: A type of somatoform disorder in which clients experience pain that has no physical basis or that exceeds the level generally expected for the level/type of injury; significant impairment of social and/or occupational functioning occurs. Two subcategories exist: *Associated with psychological factors:* The onset, severity, exacerbation, and/or maintenance of pain are significantly impacted by psychological factors; general medical conditions have no role or a minimal role in the onset. *Associated with both psychological factors and general medical condition:* Pain is due to general medical condition that is focus of presentation of symptoms and that is significant enough to warrant clinical attention; however, psychological factors impact the onset, severity, exacerbation, and/or maintenance of the pain.

· ·

Definition: A type of somatoform disorder in which client complains of multiple symptoms involving multiple organs. It stems from a severe anxiety where emotions and/or conflicts are expressed through significant multiple-system symptoms.

ALCOHOL DEPENDENCY/ABUSE

. . . .

ALCOHOL: KORSAKOFF'S PSYCHOSIS

. . . .

ALCOHOL: WERNICKE'S ENCEPHALOPATHY

Definition: Primary, chronic disease in which individual experiences impaired ability to control alcohol consumption, and/or is preoccupied with alcohol despite disruption in physical, emotional, and/or social functioning.
Causes: Combination of genetic, familial, and environmental factors.
Assessment Findings: *Dependency:* Tolerance; withdrawal symptoms when alcohol is discontinued; spending significant amount of time obtaining, drinking, or recovering from the effects of alcohol. *Abuse:* Recurrent episodes of drinking in situations where it is hazardous or where it results in the failure to fulfill obligations and/or causes alcohol-related legal problems.
Nursing Interventions: Encourage verbalization of feelings; assist client in recognition of misuse of alcohol; provide psychotherapy; refer client to Alcoholics Anonymous; encourage adherence to prescribed medication regime, including vitamin supplements; nutritional guidance.

. . . .

Definition: A type of amnesia caused by a deficiency of B complex vitamins, including thiamine and B_{12}, caused by poor nutritional habits associated with alcoholism; symptoms include disorientation, loss of short-term memory, confabulation, and inability to learn new skills.

. . . .

Definition: Degenerative condition of the brain caused by thiamine deficiency from poor nutritional intake associated with alcoholism. Symptoms include double vision, lack of coordination, decreased cognition, and involuntary/rapid eye movements.

ALCOHOL: WITHDRAWAL

....

CAGE QUESTIONNAIRE

....

NON-ALCOHOL SUBSTANCE ABUSE

PART VII

Symptoms

	Onset	Duration	Signs/Symptoms
Early Withdrawal	Hours	24 to 48 hours	Headache, anxiety, irritability, hyperalertness, sleep disturbances, shaky feeling, hand tremors, elevated heart rate, seizures (7–48 hours).
Delirium	48 to 72 hours	2 to 3 days	Agitation, anxiety, diaphoresis, disorientation, hallucinations, delusions, elevated heart rate and blood pressure, panic, vomiting, diarrhea, paranoia, coma

Nursing Interventions: Monitor vital signs, provide nonstimulating atmosphere, reorient; implement seizure precautions; stay with patient who is hallucinating; administer medications, including benzodiazepines, anticonvulsants, and thiamine as ordered.

. . . .

Definition: A screening tool for alcoholism that consists of four questions:
C: Have you ever felt that you should *cut down* on your drinking?
A: Have people *annoyed* you by criticizing your drinking?
G: Have you ever felt bad or *guilty* about your drinking?
E: Have you ever had an alcoholic drink first thing in the morning (*eye-opener*) because of a hangover, or just to get the day started?
Two positive responses to these questions indicate that further screening/ diagnostics should be completed.

. . . .

Definition: Regular use of substances that impact central nervous system functioning, resulting in behavior deviations and physiological and psychological dependence.
Causes: Combination of psychological, environmental, biological, and genetic factors.
Assessment Findings: Vary according to substance under consideration.
Nursing Interventions: Monitor vital signs, level of consciousness, electrolytes, s/s overdose/withdrawal; provide adequate rest, nutrition, and hydration; administer medications per protocol or order; confront client's denial of problem and placement of blame on others; identify stressors; assist in the development of alternative coping mechanisms.

SUBSTANCE: COCAINE

· ·

SUBSTANCE: HALLUCINOGENIC

· ·

SUBSTANCE: NARCOTICS/OPIOIDS

Overdose	Dilation of pupils, elevated blood pressure, tachycardia, cardiac arrhythmias, cardiac arrest, nausea, vomiting, diarrhea.
Withdrawal Symptoms	Apathy, irritability, confusion, prolonged periods of sleep, depression.
Special Considerations	Effect is short-lived, leading to increased use; tolerance can develop within days.

. . . .

Examples	LSD, PCP, DMT, mescaline, psilocybin mushroom.
Short-Term Effects	Increased sensory awareness and visual imagery, nausea, disrupted coordination, anxiety.
Long-Term Effects	May intensify or precipitate psychosis, panic.
Overdose	Panic, psychosis, flashbacks, impaired judgment.
Withdrawal Symptoms	No withdrawal symptoms.
Special Considerations	Protect from self-injury, reduce sensory stimuli.

. . . .

Examples	*Narcotics:* Codeine, morphine, meperidine. *Opiums:* Heroin, methadone, opium.
Short-Term Effects	Sedation, euphoria, decreased pain, impaired cognition and coordination.
Long-Term Effects	Decreased appetite, weight loss, impotency.
Overdose	Respiratory and circulatory arrest, unconsciousness, coma, death.
Withdrawal Symptoms	Watery eyes and nose, dilated pupils, diaphoresis, decreased appetite, abdominal cramps, nausea, vomiting, hallucinations, delusions, increased pulse and respirations.
Special Consideration	Narcan may reverse respiratory depression from overdose of narcotics.

SUBSTANCE: SEDATIVES

· ·

SUBSTANCE: STIMULANTS

· ·

SUBSTANCE ABUSE, IMPORTANT TERMINOLOGY

PART
VII

Examples	Barbiturates, benzodiazepines, Valium, Serax, Ativan.
Short-Term Effects	Relaxation, drowsiness, sleep induction, decreased anxiety, decreased mental alertness.
Long-Term Effects	Weight loss, irritability.
Overdose	Drowsiness, lethargy, confusion, coma, death.
Withdrawal Symptoms	Agitation, increased anxiety, sleep disturbances, seizures, depression, abdominal cramps, tremors.
Special Considerations	Treat overdose with activated charcoal/gastric lavage or Flumazenil for benzodiazepine overdose.

Examples	Benzedrine, Dexedrine, Methedrine, Ritalin.
Overdose	Increased respirations, restlessness, tremors, confusion, aggressiveness, hallucinations, panic.
Withdrawal symptoms	Depression, fatigue, hypersomnia, restlessness.
Special considerations	May develop paranoid delusions.

Term	Definition
Substance Use	Ingestion of prescription drug, over-the-counter medication, alcohol, nicotine, or illicit drug.
Dependence/Habituation	Intermittent or continuous cravings for a substance, leading to repeated use/misuse of the substance.
Tolerance	Refers to the client's ability to obtain desired effect from a substance—client requires increasing amount of substance to obtain desired effect.
Withdrawal	Clinical symptoms produced from a cessation in the use of a substance.

THERAPEUTIC COMMUNICATION, PHASES OF

. . . .

THERAPEUTIC COMMUNICATION TECHNIQUES, I

. . . .

PART VII

Initiating/Orienting	Nurse sets stage by ensuring privacy and begins to build trust and rapport; assessment of needs and communication preferences is conducted; therapeutic contracts are established.
Working Phase	Discussion conducted on mutually set goals; identification of coping mechanisms, perceptions, and supports occurs; alternative behaviors are explored.
Termination Phase	Identification of progress and need for further referrals is conducted; when goals have been met, the nurse ends the relationship; it is not unusual for clients to exhibit anxiety or regression during this phase and may attempt to prolong the relationship; planning for the termination of the relationship should begin during the initiation stage.

Acknowledgment	Recognition of client's effort, behavior, and/or communication. Example: "I noticed that you initiated the conversation today."
Clarification	Used to ensure understanding of client's statement(s). Example: "I am not sure of what you are saying."
Focusing	Helping client to concentrate on or expand on a given topic. Example: "It appears that you are worried about losing your job."
Giving Information	Presenting factual information. Example: "You may feel drowsy with this medication."
Offering of Self	Being present with client. Example: "I will stay with you during the procedure."
Open-Ended Questions/Statements	Questions/statements that encourage client to provide more than a yes/no answer. Example: "Tell me about the argument."

THERAPEUTIC COMMUNICATION TECHNIQUES, II

Paraphrasing	Repeating back to client his or her underlying thoughts or feelings. Example: "You felt sad when your daughter stated she was moving."
Presentation of Reality	Assisting the client in differentiating the real from the unreal. Example: "I do not see that."
Reflecting	Directing clients' thoughts or feelings back to them for further exploration. Example: "You seem unsure about telling your daughter."
Silence	Being quiet with client without interrupting any pauses or breaks in the conversation, thereby allowing client time to collect thoughts/feelings.
Touch	Touching client in an appropriate, culturally sensitive manner to convey caring attitude.

BEHAVIORAL THERAPY

. . . .

COGNITIVE THERAPY

. . . .

CRISIS INTERVENTION

PART
VII

Definition: Treatment modality that utilizes learning principles to effect changes in behavior by focusing on the consequences of actions; undesirable actions are viewed as learned behaviors that can be modified.

. . . .

Definition: Short-term treatment modality that focuses on replacing client's negative or irrational beliefs and/or distorted attitude; delivered in group or individual setting; client's cognitive abilities must not be impaired for modality to be effective; utilizes problem-solving to identify and overcome issues.

. . . .

Definition: Treatment modality focused on resolution of crisis situation that the client is unable to handle alone; utilizes identification of immediate coping patterns with a goal of returning client to precrisis level of functioning; generally six weeks in duration or less.

FAMILY THERAPY

. . . .

GROUP THERAPY

. . . .

MILIEU THERAPY

PART
VII

Definition: A modality that utilizes the client's family versus the individual client as the focus for therapy; utilizes family system theory to assess the functioning of the family and the client within the family to identify members, roles, life scripts, self-fulfilling prophecies, and incongruent communications; goal is to decrease conflict and promote appropriate family functionality and interrelationships.

• •

Definition: Treatment modality that involves two or more clients and one or more healthcare professionals interacting to resolve emotional or self-esteem issues and improve behavior and social functioning; members test reality by giving and receiving feedback.

• •

Definition: Treatment is provided through the planned use of the treatment environment, including people, resources, and activities. It includes everyone who comes into contact with the client. Focuses on activities, limit setting, and client decision making, and allows for the testing of situations in a realistic way through the provision of a microcosm of the outside environment.

ACETYLCHOLINESTERONE INHIBITORS

· ·

ANTIPARKINSON

· ·

ANTIPSYCHOTIC

Example Medications	Donnepezil (Aricept), galantamine (Reminyl), tacrine (Cognex).
Use	Treatment of Alzheimer's disease.
Adverse Reactions	Nausea, diarrhea, elevated liver enzymes.
Nursing Implications	Contraindicated with anticholinergic medications; medication should not be abruptly discontinued.

. . . .

Example Medications	Artane, Cogentin, Kemadrin, Akineton.
Use	Treatment of extrapyramidal symptoms from antipsychotic medications.
Adverse Reactions	Vertigo, urinary hesitation, GI distress, disruption in cognition.

. . . .

Example Medications	Thorazine, Stelazine, Trilafon, Prolixin, Haldol, Clozaril, Loxitane.
Use	Relief of psychotic symptoms; behavioral control.
Adverse Reactions	Extrapyramidal symptoms: *Drug-induced Parkinson:* Shuffling gait, tremors, pill-rolling movement, dyskinesia, flat affect. *Akathesia:* Uncontrolled restlessness, toe tapping, pacing. *Dystonia:* Spasms of neck and limbs, disruption of coordination. *Tardive dyskinesia:* Permanent gait shuffling, drooling, dystonia. Hypotension, increased liver enzymes, dry mouth, blurred vision, tachycardia, constipation.
Nursing Implications	Monitor for *neuroleptic malignant syndrome*: rigidity; irregular/erratic pulse, blood pressure, respirations; change in mental status; elevated creatinine; if present, stop medication and administer dopamine as ordered.

ANTI-SUBSTANCE ABUSE

. . . .

ATYPICAL ANTIDEPRESSANTS

. . . .

BARBITURATES/SEDATIVES

PART VII

Example Medication	Disulfiram (Antabuse).
Use	Assists client to stop drinking alcohol by causing the client to experience negative symptoms if alcohol is consumed while on the medication.
Adverse Reactions	Occur if alcohol is consumed while taking medication, and include nausea, vomiting, throbbing headache, vertigo, blurred vision, thirst, confusion, diaphoresis.
Nursing Implications	Ensure client understands the adverse effect of alcohol consumption while on the medication; does not prevent withdrawal symptoms.

• •

Example Medications	Wellbutrin, Remeron, Nefazodone, Trazodone.
Use	Treatment of depression.
Adverse Reactions	Vary according to medication. *Wellbutrin:* Anxiety, restlessness, sleep disturbances, dry mouth, agitation, headache, sore throat, tremors. *Remeron:* Increased appetite, increased cholesterol; changes in blood pressure, decreased white blood cells, weight gain. *Nefazodone:* Blurred vision, vertigo, dry mouth, headache, nausea, weakness, sleeplessness, decreased blood pressure. *Trazodone:* Nausea, diarrhea, constipation, confusion, arrhythmia, confusion, headache, dry mouth.
Nursing Implications	Monitor for signs and symptoms of suicide, especially as client's energy and mood increase.

• •

Example Medications	*Barbiturates:* Amytal Sodium, Butisol Sodium, Nembutal Sodium, Seconal Sodium, Luminal Sodium. *Sedatives:* Aquachloral Supprettes, Lunesta, Miltown, Roxerem, Sonata, Ambien.
Use	Treatment of anxiety, sleep disorders.
Adverse Reactions	Drowsiness, confusion, lethargy, hangover effect, megaloblastic anemia, thrombocytopenic purpura, agranulocytosis.
Nursing Implications	Client to avoid alcohol, avoid driving or operating heavy machinery; patient should take medication 30 minutes prior to bedtime if using for insomnia; client should not stop medication abruptly.

BENZODIAZEPINES

. . . .

MONOAMINE OXIDASE INHIBITORS (MAOIs)

. . . .

PART
VII

Example Medications	Xanax, Librium, Klonopin, Tranxene, Valium, Ativan, Versed, Serax, Restoril, Halcion.
Use	Treatment of anxiety.
Adverse Reactions	Daytime drowsiness, vertigo, headaches, blurred vision, hypotension, incontinence, amnesia, slurred speech, lethargy. *Toxicity:* Somnolence, confusion, decreased reflexes, coma.
Nursing Implications	Elderly clients are at risk of falling. Client should avoid use of alcohol. Cessation of medication can cause withdrawal symptoms. Toxicity can be reversed with IV administration of flumazenil (Romazicon).

Example Medications	Marplan, Nardil, Parnate.
Use	Treatment of depression.
Adverse Reactions	Orthostatic hypotension, insomnia, lethargy, dry mouth, increased weight, edema, anxiety, agitation, mania, headaches, constipation, impotence.
Nursing Implications	Drug interaction with sympathomimetic medications and/or foods containing tyramine* may cause hypertensive crisis: hypertension, radiating headache, nausea and vomiting, change in mental status, chest pain, chills, stiff neck; treatment of choice for hypertensive crisis is IV phentolamine (Regitine).

*Tyramine-containing foods include avocados, bananas, liver, caffeine, aged cheese, figs, meat tenderizers, overripe fruits, papayas, raisins, red wine, beer, sherry, salami, sausage, pepperoni, bologna, sour cream, soy sauce, yogurt.

MOOD STABILIZERS/ANTIMANIC

. . . .

SELECTIVE SEROTONIN REUPTAKE
INHIBITORS (SSRIs)

. . . .

Example Medication	Lithium.
Use	Control of mood disorders.
Adverse Reactions	Polyuria, polydipsia, anorexia, dry mouth, increased weight, bloating, fatigue, headache, hair loss, diarrhea, metallic taste. *Toxicity:* Blood level exceeds 1.5 to 2.0 mEq/L; symptoms include nausea, vomiting, tremors, slurred speech, twitching, oliguria.
Nursing Implications	Therapeutic range 0.6 to 1.2 mEq/L; monitor sodium intake; client should consume normal dietary intake, sodium deficiency increases risk for toxicity; toxicity is managed via administration of mannitol, gastric lavage, and management of fluid and electrolytes.

Example Medications	Celexa, Lexapro, Prozac, Luvox, Paxil, Prexeva, Zoloft.
Use	Treatment of depression.
Adverse Reactions	Nausea, drowsiness, anxiety, sleep disturbances, headache, vertigo, seizures, changes in weight, apathy, tremors, diaphoresis, dry mouth.
Nursing Implications	Monitor BP, assess for suicide. Avoid use with monoamine oxidase inhibitors. Prozac in combination with other SSRIs can be fatal; when changing medications, need 5-week space between Prozac and other SSRI due to long half-life of Prozac. Avoid abrupt discontinuation of medication. There may be increased bleeding with use of NSAIDs. Client education includes avoidance of over-the-counter cold medicines, and taking care to change positions slowly.

TRICYCLIC ANTIDEPRESSANTS

Example Medications	Amitryptyline, Aventyl, Elavil, Norpramin, Pamelor, Sinequan, Surmontil, Tofranil, Vivactil.
Use	Treatment of depression.
Adverse Reactions	Dry mouth, blurred vision, postural hypotension, constipation, arrhythmias, sedation, weight gain, irritability, anxiety, photosensitivity. *Overdose:* Arrhythmias, agitation, flushing, pupil dilation, seizures, hallucinations, coma.
Nursing Implications	Assess for suicide risk; client education includes taking medication as prescribed, checking with healthcare provider prior to taking over-the-counter cold medications to avoid drug interaction, and avoiding use of alcohol.
Special Considerations	If client's medication is changed to a monoamine oxidase inhibitor, 1 to 3 weeks should elapse between medications to avoid hypertensive crisis.

ADDITIONAL ONLINE PRACTICE

Whether you need help building basic skills or preparing for an exam, visit LearningExpress Practice Center! Using the code below, you'll be able to access additional online NCLEX-RN practice. This online practice will also provide you with:

Immediate scoring
Detailed answer explanations
A customized diagnostic report that will assess your skills and focus your study

Log in to the LearningExpress Practice Center by using the URL: **www.learnatest.com/practice**

This is your Access Code: **8936**

Follow the steps online to redeem your access code. After you've used your access code to register with the site, you will be prompted to create a username and password. For easy reference, record them here:

Username: _____ **Password:** _____

If you have any questions or problems, please contact LearningExpress customer service at 1-800-295-9556 ext. 2, or e-mail us at **customerservice@learningexpressllc.com**

NOTES

NOTES